Weight Control
for a Young America

Weight Control
for a Young America

Happy, Healthy Kids
Who Eat Right from Wrong

by Keith Klein

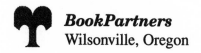

BookPartners
Wilsonville, Oregon

W

The recommendations in this book are not substitutes or replacements for clinical consultations or evaluations. Before starting your child on any weight loss program, please consult a physician for advice. Some of the products and food labels discussed here may have changed since printing of this book. Therefore, please check the label of any product cited before making a decision to purchase it.

Table of Contents

Introduction

The best way to reduce obesity in America is to start with our children. Overweight children grow into overweight adults. Obesity is usually a family affair, because kids tend to copy their parents' eating habits as well as their lifestyle. Fortunately, the road to better health and weight control is quite simple. If we can teach our kids to eat better and become more active, many of the hardships they would otherwise face in the future from being overweight can be alleviated.

Weight Control for a Young America is dedicated to every child and parent who desires to embark on a lifetime of sound nutrition and good health. Now there is solid proof that heart disease begins early in life but may not show up until years later. What your child eats today will have a definite impact on his or her health tomorrow. This book has been written for all parents, not just those with overweight kids, and it will show you how to prevent high blood pressure, diabetes, and elevated cholesterol or triglyceride levels and keep your kids healthy. Prevention is the best way to circumvent future problems. Don't wait until your son or daughter has a health or weight problem to start on a program that will improve the quality of his or her life.

If your child is already overweight or obese, be encouraged: There are solid answers to your questions and appropriate ways to help resolve the issues. You are taking an important step to restore balance in his or her life by reading this book. It is designed to help you help your child overcome weight problems. If you have "tried everything" without success and are tempted to give in, remember, hopelessness and helplessness are nothing more than a perceived lack of solutions. *Weight Control for a Young America* provides new solutions that have been proven to work.

Without realizing it, you may be one of those parents who pass along your own weight-related fears and dieting behaviors to your children. A mother who is overly concerned about her own weight may unintentionally convey her anxiety to her kids. To prevent this, we must become aware of the messages that we consciously or unconsciously pass on to our children.

Believe it or not, there is no such thing as a truly independent self-image. Our self-perception, every thought and feeling we have about ourselves, is formed early in life by the reflections we get back from those around us. In childhood, our parents, siblings, and others with whom we associate act as mirrors that reflect back to us a sense of wholeness and identity.

As a parent, what you reflect to your child confirms or undermines her image of herself. Statements such as "I love you," "You're special to me," "You're so smart," or

"You're the greatest kid a parent could ever hope for" contribute to her positive sense of identity. If a child is lucky, she'll get thousands of messages that tell her she's loved and special.

Unfortunately, negative comments like "Don't you have anything better to do?" "You're such a slob," "Why can't you be more like your sister?" are direct attacks on a child's sense of worth. She may try to compensate by using food to offset her feelings of unworthiness. It is important for you to project the right attitude to your daughter before you can expect to see changes in her behavior.

Focus on unconditional acceptance of your daughter, *as she is*. Consciously and deliberately choose a positive way to make your point. Explain to your daughter, for example, that your family is going to move toward healthier eating "because it's good for all of us," not "because you're fat."

Regardless of your son's body shape or physical condition, positive reinforcement from you maximizes his self-esteem and helps him to feel good emotionally and physically. Positive mirroring—reflection of approval from you—is the most important foundation on which to build his self-esteem and help him overcome his weight problem.

Mirroring doesn't end in childhood. As we move out into the adult world we continually receive images from other people that tell us how we look, act and sound. Although the parents may be good mirrors, the rest of the world may be projecting stronger negative messages. Overweight children are often the butt of jokes, ridicule, teasing and cruel laughter from other youngsters. The mirror image that reaches out to them from their peers is one of being fat and unworthy. Overweight children are influenced by direct and indirect mirror messages or disapproval, innuendo, body language, and facial expressions. And although overweight children may be bashful and ashamed of their bodies, they cannot conceal their problem from other kids. They constantly compare themselves to their slimmer counterparts at the pool, the park, the playground, wherever kids play and socialize.

As a parent, you must persist in reflecting unconditional love and acceptance to your kids, and never resort to criticism about their weight. With a solid sense of identity and high self-esteem, your child will be equipped to learn how to assess the responses of others and to understand that there is a profound difference between someone's opinion, mindless criticism, and fact. Consistent, openly expressed approval from parents builds into a child a strong *self*-approval that is not easily shaken.

Be Careful of the Messages You Send
Several years ago, while working with teenagers who had eating disorders, I noticed similarities between many of them. Somewhere along the line, these kids received messages that they were fat, even though they weren't, and most of their eating disorders surfaced after they failed at numerous attempts to lose weight on their own.

I have one particularly poignant recollection of a fifteen-year-old girl who told me about her first memory of feeling fat and unattractive. Lauren had spent an entire afternoon shopping for an evening gown to wear to a party with her family. She was so excited about looking glamorous in her new dress that she could hardly wait to surprise her parents. She spent the whole afternoon doing her hair, nails and makeup. When her parents called her to come downstairs, Lauren made a grand entrance from the top of the stairs. To her dismay, neither her mom or dad complimented her on her appearance—not a single word.

When the family climbed into the car, Mom finally told Lauren how nice she looked. "But," she added, "you would look like an angel if you were just ten pounds lighter." In truth, Lauren wasn't fat or ugly, but her mother's single deflating statement became the principal message that Lauren replayed to herself from then on. Feeling unlovable and overweight, she battled ongoing discouragement, always trying the latest diet, which she hoped would make her thin and more attractive.

What Can You Expect from This Program?

When you understand the correct methods to help your child develop a lifelong healthy relationship with food, and learn how to build her self-esteem, your sense of hope-lessness and helplessness will be eliminated. If your daughter feels sensitive about her body image or is being teased about her weight, you will learn in this book how to approach her concerns without making matters worse. Also, you will discover how to teach her to avoid developing a dieter's mentality. By following the step-by-step program displayed in the following pages, and showing your daughter the way, not only will she lose unwanted pounds but she will also develop a more positive attitude and better body image.

As a caring parent, you have to understand the issues involved in nutrition and weight loss if you wish to help your children lose weight successfully. Incorrect informa-tion from you, or the wrong attitude, can cause them a great deal of harm, both mentally and metabolically, for the rest of their lives. That's why it is so important for you to under-stand the issues and subtleties of a positive weight control program that can guide your children not only through successful weight loss, but to the establishment of a supportive mental image of themselves. It can serve as the compass that will lead them to positive growth and maturity.

How Fast Will My Child Lose Unwanted Pounds?

It's important to point out that a weight problem cannot be resolved in a week. You should not be looking for an overnight quick fix or a fad diet. *Weight Control for a Young America* is designed to provide you with the tools to help your child, to show him where his proper focus should be to reach a long-term destination. The major focus must be on changing and developing lifelong nutritional habits, not on how much and how fast your child can lose weight. Your child's weight is not the problem, it is a symptom and a by-product of other problems, such as too much snacking, not enough activity, and poor food choices.

The best and only reliable way to treat overweight children is to *reduce their fat and sugar intake, increase their physical activity, decrease their television watching, and let them grow into their weight*. This book shows how to make simple changes that lead to big differences.

It's Not Just a Book

Children and adults alike will enjoy the recipes that are located in the back of the book. In addition to simple, low fat recipes, there are ideas on how you can modify many of your family's current favorite high fat recipes.

Not to worry—snacks and desserts are part of a healthy eating program. Healthy eating is not about deprivation. It is about eating the wrong kinds of foods in moderation.

A Note About Style

Obesity can affect both boys and girls, but to avoid endless repetition of "he/she" and "him/her" and the awkwardness of such gender-neutral terms as "your child," I have opted simply to alternate between male and female references throughout the book. The examples given and the remedies suggested apply equally to boys or girls.

Short and Sweet Summary

Here is a quick preview of the major points to be presented, to prepare you for what lies ahead.

1. *Weight Control for a Young America* is not about fostering weight loss for your child. It introduces a method of healthy eating for life.
2. A child's weight on the bathroom scale is not an indicator of success but rather an arbitrary number that does more harm than good. You must keep your child off the scale.
3. Exercise is one of the most important indicators of lifetime health and weight control.
4. Arm yourself with nutritional knowledge. You are the best advocate for your own family.
5. Weight loss, as defined here, is not about a quick fix or a fad diet, but about changing behaviors that will result in weight loss and improved attitudes about food.
6. Better Bad Choices™* allow a child to develop the decision-making process.
7. Nutritious nibbling increases a child's metabolism and helps to prevent potential bingeing. Let your child eat nutritious snacks between meals.

8. Deprivation leads to nothing but problems.
9. Be creative both in food preparation and in structuring time.
10. Good habits, which can always be learned, enable children to be in control of their food and, by extension, more in control of themselves.

The program presented here isn't one you should try to digest, so to speak, in one sitting. Rather, I advise you to read small sections and take your time to comprehend the materials properly. As you read each section, think about developing your own plan and tailor the recommendations from the section to fit the needs of your family.

Chapter 1

Where Did This Weight Gain Come From?

"Mommy, am I fat?" is typically an innocent question, but the way you respond could make all the difference in the world to your son. Your son may be slightly bigger than other children his age for various reasons, including skeletal size (frame or muscle size), or excess body weight. In any case, your first response should be to find out why your son is asking this question. Perhaps another child in the neighborhood prompted it by name-calling, or maybe your son heard the teasing of a boy or girl with a body shape similar to his. Maybe his brother or sister did the taunting, or your son may have heard you talk about your weight problem long enough to pick up your insecurity and apply it to himself. No matter how his question came about, you must approach the answer carefully. If you agree and tell your son that he is fat, he may live with that label for a lifetime.

In many cases, when a child is insecure about his weight or shape, the condition isn't overweight at all, but may be the result of his parents labeling the child as fat because they have misidentified their son's basic body structure. It doesn't look like their own, they complain, not thinking that the boy may have inherited a grandparent's genes! Thin mothers have brought their daughters to me with such statements as, "But she's not fitting into her clothes," or "She's only fifteen years old, she shouldn't weigh 130 pounds." Messages like these convince a girl that something is wrong with her and her body. If Mom were not so concerned, the daughter would be fine.

Let's begin by distinguishing between weight gain from poor dietary habits and weight gain from growing bones and muscles.

Hormones versus Habits

Your fourteen-year-old daughter comes home one day crying because she feels fat. Secretly, you've been concerned because you have noticed that she's put on a few pounds. She has added two clothing sizes in three months so you know her extra weight gain is not a figment of your imagination. To comfort her, you sympathize, pointing out that you've been down that road yourself. To support her plan to lose weight, you and she start on a diet regimen of lettuce, cabbage soup and removal of all the junk food from the pantry. Without realizing it, you have started your daughter on a lifetime struggle with her body image and weight. It will only get harder for her to fight the battle of the bulge as she grows older.

What many a well-intentioned mother doesn't understand is that her daughter may not need a diet at all. She may require an explanation of basic human physiology. The fact is, some weight gain is due to hormonal changes, not poor eating habits. Most childhood weight gain is a natural result of the growth process. What actually takes place is a hormonal flux that happens to all children. It's hard to predict exactly at what age your child may experience hormonal change, because all children mature and develop at different ages.

In the case of the girl described above, her body probably has begun to release the female hormone estrogen. Estrogen is responsible for female characteristics such as a supple body, breast development, and soft skin. During adolescence, excess estrogen causes the same physiological responses that all women experience during their menstrual cycle: food cravings, water retention, weight gain—sound familiar? Dieting at this time may hinder physical development and lead to physiological problems as well as psychological problems with food.

Because girls do gain a little bit of body fat during this stage of development, it's very easy to understand how a parent can interpret these changes as a weight gain resulting from eating rather than the normal course of development, but all kids experience weight gain simply because they are in a perpetual state of growth from birth until their early twenties. They don't have to get taller or appear fat to gain weight. Bones are becoming denser, muscles are getting larger, organs are growing, and various water compartments shift during hormonal fluxes. An adolescent girl can retain excess water and appear to gain weight. Likewise, she can dehydrate, lose body water, and appear to lose weight. In both cases, even though her actual body weight remains the same, the fluctuations in water content may cause the bathroom scale to register a gain or a loss, much to the girl's horror or delight.

With boys, the story is the same, but with a different twist. In many cases, the baby fat a boy carries may result from a lack of the male hormone, testosterone. Testosterone is responsible for male characteristics such as large muscles, low body fat, and facial hair.

Most boys experience a growth spurt about the age of fourteen or fifteen, although some carry their baby fat a little longer. During this time of sudden growth, many boys shed fat, gain muscle, and grow taller. But if your son's hormonal changes are delayed, he may carry baby fat longer and appear overweight. In some cases, a deficiency of testosterone may be the root cause of excess body fat, lack of sexual development, and the appearance of breast tissue. If by age sixteen your son appears underdeveloped, simple blood chemistry and hormonal tests by a physician can determine whether his excess weight is due to a testosterone deficiency.

Once again, just because your child carries a little extra body fat, don't react by putting him on a diet. Growing kids need lots of food and nutrients. It's perfectly normal for growth spurts to speed up or slow down. Consequently, your son may become pudgy during one stage and too thin during another. These weight changes and fluctuations are common but many parents react too quickly, which in turn creates more problems for the growing child.

Body Types

Recent studies have concluded that an individual's body size and shape are genetically coded. A child's skeletal structure, metabolic rate, and distribution of body fat are programmed through the genes passed down by the parents. Body shape and body size are predetermined and inherited, like hair color, eye color, or the shape of a nose. Consequently, despite many attempts to lose weight over the course of life, some people just can't seem to get thin. Furthermore, these heredity factors overwhelm other factors that normally determine a person's range of body weight. Although diet and exercise play an important role in determining a person's weight, they seem to do so within the limits set by heredity. Most people demonstrate a fairly stable "normal" weight, which is one reason why many of us return to our original weight when we complete a diet that doesn't include regular exercise.

Structural Differences
There are three distinct classifications of the human body: mesomorph, endomorph and ectomorph. Your child will fall into one of these three categories.

Mesomorph
A mesomorph tends to be muscular and well-defined, with a low percentage of body fat. Children who possess this type of body structure tend to be naturals at sports such as football or wrestling. Imagine Arnold Schwarzenegger, Mary Lou Retton or Jackie Joyner-Kersee and you will get the picture!

Ectomorph

Children with ectomorphic physiques are usually very skinny. They are the ones who can eat anything and everything and never put on pounds. In fact, gaining weight for an ectomorph can be as difficult as losing weight is for someone who is overweight. Ectomorphs tend to be good at sports such as tennis, running, or basketball. Although Don Knotts and Twiggy may seem an unlikely pair, they both have ectomorphic builds.

Endomorph

Endomorphs are pear-shaped. They tend to gain weight easily and struggle with their figures. Examples of these athletes are sumo wrestlers or football linemen. Oprah Winfrey and Rosie O'Donnell have more in common than talk shows—both are endomorphs. If your child has a weight problem, chances are he has this type of physique. But don't give up hope! I have a solution.

You Can Overcome Your Child's Basic Structure

I used to be very skinny, an ectomorph. Today, I'm 205 pounds with 5 percent body fat. My best friend has twin brothers, endomorphs who struggle with their weight. At one time they both weighed the same. One brother now weighs almost 300 pounds; the other is 176 pounds with 10 percent body fat. How did these genetic body shapes change? I'm still an ectomorph and the twins are still endomorphs, but the difference lies in our exercise habits. Weight lifting allowed me to put more muscle on my body. Jogging allowed the thin brother to keep his weight under control but the heavier one is a couch potato. That's why it's important to get your child involved in a regular exercise program. Exercise is a great way for your child to modify her body's response to its genetic coding.

Chapter 2

Measures of Success

<hr>

The Damage of Frequent Weighing

Don't Allow Your Child to Step on the Scale

Have you ever felt great about your own eating and exercise programs only to jump onto a scale and discover a two pound weight gain instead of the three pound weight loss you were expecting? Imagine what it's like for your child. Your daughter may not be old enough to understand the difference between good weight gain and bad. In her eyes, the upward movement of the scale is always bad. And a slight increase in your daughter's weight may cause you to make unnecessary adjustments in her eating program. A further decrease in food intake may lead to cravings and a lingering greater preoccupation with certain foods. Within a few short weeks, she could end up bingeing, gaining more weight in fat, and feeling like a failure.

Frequent weighing actually encourages the very same compulsive tendencies that we want to cure in your child. A scale is a useful tool for marking and charting progress, but it shouldn't be used as a sole indicator of success. Does this mean a child should never be weighed? No, but perhaps we can look at the numbers creatively. Show your daughter how far she has come rather than how far she still has to go. For example, let's say she weighs 135 and a good weight for her would be 120. Rather than telling her that she has fifteen pounds to lose, let her know that she is only five pounds away from the 120 range. Five pounds seems easy enough to reach. Pretty soon, she will be in the 120s. And once she's there, she will be only eight or nine pounds away from her goal. I have found that this approach builds a child's confidence, because the goal becomes tangible—and not as far away as imagined.

Don't Allow an Inanimate Object to Have Power over Your Child's Life

As I've indicated, the bathroom scale is not a good indicator of how well a child is progressing toward his goal. It gives significance to an arbitrary number that doesn't consider bone structure, genetics, or other individual factors.

Years ago, while working with bulimia and anorexia clients, I realized that their disorder was strongly tied to the scale. In fact, one criterion used to determine whether a girl had an eating disorder was how often she weighed herself. Weighing often indicates how strongly preoccupied a girl is with her body image.

If your daughter is trying her best to lose weight but the scale doesn't go down fast enough, she may get frustrated and angry. Even after she is able to wear a smaller clothing size, the scale may not reflect the loss dramatically enough to satisfy her or you. Weighing can cause tension and increased feelings of failure. Weighing a child is a lot like competition for the best grade or most expensive outfit. It becomes a basis of comparison by which your child will quickly learn to compare herself to other kids. As children get taller, their bones become denser, and muscle mass increases—all good things—and their weight will fluctuate. Even though your daughter's weight is increasing, her body fat percentage could be decreasing—a great accomplishment!

How Crazy Can the Scale Make Your Child?

If it seems that I dwell on the problems of overusing the scale, it is because I have seen how destructive reliance on it can be to the weight-reducing aspirations of kids. The scale can lead to very dichotomous thinking. Dichotomous thinkers have strong, one-sided viewpoints concerning particular topics, which are the basis for an all-or-nothing attitude. Dichotomous thinkers see no gray areas, only black or white. In many cases, this type of reasoning causes your child to overgeneralize problems; only failures seem to matter. The child who develops black-or-white reasoning usually measures her self-worth by errors and weaknesses rather than by strengths and successes.

A child who weighs frequently is continually receiving feedback that leads to defeating, negative self-talk. He will forget about any progress he has made, because all of his past accomplishments have become worthless compared to the magnitude of one slight increase on the scale. Like a steel ball on a pendulum, caught oscillating between two magnets, your son becomes engrossed in dichotomous thinking, swinging between satisfaction and disappointment, unable to settle for gradual progress.

A negative weigh-in, or one that doesn't live up to your son's expectations, can trigger bingeing. If the scale doesn't respond the way your son expects, he may decide that eating correctly and exercising simply are not worth the sacrifice. It can be the first in a series of dominoes that begin to fall, leading to a relapse. What child (or adult, for that matter) wants to keep doing something that makes him feel like a failure?

You Should Question the Very Idea of Dieting

For many of us, the journey toward health begins with the pursuit of thinness. The full-length mirror doesn't lie. One day, when we are feeling very brave, we decide to look at ourselves critically in this mirror. Often we become slightly disgusted with what we see. "Well," we say, "it's easy enough to change things." We attempt to make changes in our diet by slashing calories and promising ourselves to start exercising or perhaps exercise more than we already do. We believe that by eating less, we can reach our ideal body shape.

Surprise: Without realizing it, our approach may lead to even more problems. Most people don't realize that the approaches they implement to lose weight are the very ones that cause them to become increasingly heavier with each passing year. In fact, the very idea of dieting has come into question after decades of thinking that strict calorie restriction, low carbohydrate diets, and liquid protein diets are the way to go. Contrary to the wishes many people have, there is no magic pill or gimmick that will solve a weight problem.

Americans are fatter and weigh more today than ever before. Adult obesity is more prevalent in America than in any other country. Americans responded in 1993 by spending twenty-five billion dollars on diets and diet-related products. Fifty million Americans are dieting at any given time, and it's safe to say that most of them are very confused. On average, those who *lose weight fast* gain back all of the weight, and more, within three years.

It's no great shock that the average American child is heavier than that in any other country. Our kids are bombarded every morning, afternoon, and night with commercials touting the fun of eating bowls of cereal, chips, and ice cream. Ninety-one percent of the foods advertised to children on television are high in fat, sugar, and/or salt, according to California researchers who assessed commercials aired during children's programs on six major networks. Other researchers have shown that children's food requests are linked to the number of hours they watch television each week. Yet another group of researchers recently reported that the number of overweight children and adolescents in the United States has more than doubled since the 1960s.

Not the Weigh to Go!

Let's look at some of the inappropriate ways parents might decide to help their child shed unwanted weight.

Weight Loss Clinics

The weight loss clinics create advertising that appears trustworthy. They offer hope to potential clients that their special product or service can make them thin regardless of how overweight they are. They often use pictures that show remarkable progress, such as a client who lost one hundred pounds or more. However, they fail to mention that extreme weight loss is the exception, not the rule.

Be careful about taking your child or yourself to a weight loss chain. In the battle for the weight loss dollar, there are many people and companies that claim they alone have a special knowledge, skill, or hidden secret that will help you or your child overcome the weight problem. And their message usually includes the words *quick, fast,* or *easy.* The commercials and advertisements make weight loss look easy and everlasting, and claim that it's possible without exercising or cutting calories. They use terms like breakthrough, miraculous, astounding, or sensational. Unfortunately, in most cases, these messages are just advertising *hype.* There are no easy, magic potions, and losing weight permanently requires dietary and lifestyle changes.

Also, beware of products that suggest that they contain a certain food, combination of foods, or supplements with a magical property to help you lose weight. (Run—don't walk—away from this one.) Unless a well-balanced, low fat eating plan is suggested, avoid the weight loss centers. Instead, go to a nutritionist or dietician who specializes in dietary programs for children. But keep one thing in mind: your child doesn't need to see the specialist—you do. Taking your child in is rarely necessary.

Liquid Diets

Don't ever allow your child or teenager to be put on a liquid protein fast. It is one of the worst things you can do. Liquid protein diets will ruin a child's chances of ever having a normal metabolism again. More important, a liquid diet will also have long-lasting emotional effects concerning food.

Diet companies and products that are cleverly advertised to offer healthy and nutritious ways to help people lose weight may actually do more harm than good. During the 1970s and 1980s, there were approximately sixty deaths resulting from liquid protein diets. In the 1980s, a number of deaths occurred among persons using one liquid diet powder. The problem with liquid diets is that they can result in a loss of muscle, and because the heart is a muscle, any loss of body protein can result in heart failure. However, it is nearly impossible to trace, much less prove, a diet-related death. It's so easy to blame the cardiac arrest on the fact that the person was overweight as opposed to undernourished. These products should never be given to a child. A liquid diet isn't normal; it exposes a child to deprivation.

Many still don't understand the dangers I've described. Current retail sales of popular, poorly designed meal replacements are better than ever. Can a concoction of milk, water, sugar, and oil, with vitamins stirred in, and eating one balanced meal per day be safe or effective? The typical "weight loss" liquid meal contains sugar (dextrose, sucrose, corn syrup, or fructose) and lots of it! Furthermore, these weight loss products are normally loaded with fat, artificial colors, and artificial flavors. These are not suitable products for anyone, especially children. The bottom line: Real food and nutritious snacks, coupled with more activity, are the best way to help your child lose weight and keep it off.

Why You Don't Want Your Child to Diet

How a Child Becomes a Deceptive, Guilty Eater

Rachel developed what she considered a weight problem. So she and her mother decided to go on a diet together. They agreed on certain bad foods to be avoided as well as good ones to eat. And they threw away all the junk food. Sounds like a perfect plan, right?

But as time progressed, Rachel saw her family members and friends eating those forbidden foods and a little resentment began to build. One day, Rachel was at a birthday party with lots of her friends. Everyone was singing "Happy Birthday" and eating cake, when that perfect combination of cake and icing was passed to her. Not wanting to appear different, Rachel ate the cake. It tasted so good that she ate two or three more slices. As she licked the last bit of icing off her lips, Rachel was overcome with guilt. She had violated the rules she and her mother set out to follow when they began their diet. However, a sneaky thought occurred to Rachel: Because nobody (meaning Mom) saw her eat the cake, it's okay. Rachel's thinking was typical of two major characteristics that plague dieters: guilty eating and deceptive eating. Both of these patterns can last a lifetime. As I discuss later, guilt and deception are two potentially dangerous outcomes that can be prevented.

How Dieting Can Stunt Your Child's Growth

Your son has put on a lot of weight very suddenly so you decide it should be taken off quickly as well. "Come on," you reason with him, "if you eat healthy foods like salads, fruits, vegetables, and rice cakes, you will lose the weight fast and then you can eat the good stuff again." Better yet, your son loves cabbage, and you have discovered the Cabbage Soup Diet in a national magazine. You assume that because the diet appears in a well-known magazine such as the *Celebrity Gazette*, it must be safe or it wouldn't be printed. Unfortunately, the diet lacks enough sustenance for a growing boy. The calories are a lot lower than they should be, not enough protein is being consumed, and essential vitamins and minerals are missing. Strict diets, not just liquid diets, often result in a loss of muscle as well as fat. It has been estimated that for every ten pounds of weight one loses on a strict diet, between four and six pounds may be lost from muscle. Losing muscle mass is bad because when muscle is lost, the body's metabolic rate slows down and fewer calories are burned. We will explore this in more detail in the following example.

The Yo-Yo Syndrome

You have probably heard about yo-yo dieting. This occurs when a person keeps losing and regaining the same fifty pounds over and over again. Down and up, down and up. What most parents don't understand is that there are other problems that dieting can create for their kids. Let's take Rachel, put her on a strict diet, and watch what the outcome produces over a short period of time.

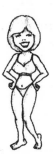

STEP 1: Rachel weighs 90 pounds and has 18 percent body fat, which is a normal weight and body fat percentage for her age and height. Let's break down her body composition and separate her fat weight from her lean body mass.

16.2 pounds of Rachel's weight are fat
73.8 pounds of her weight are lean body mass

STEP 2: Rachel goes away to camp during the summer and eats lots of candy and junk food, gaining twenty pounds of fat. As expected, her body composition changes. She now weighs 110 pounds and is 32.9 percent fat, too heavy for her height and age.

Once again, let's look at her body composition from the first example and compare it to her new body composition.

36.2 pounds of Rachel's weight are fat
73.8 pounds are still lean body mass

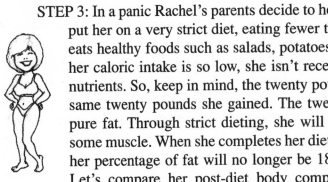

STEP 3: In a panic Rachel's parents decide to help her shed the weight quickly. They put her on a very strict diet, eating fewer than nine hundred calories a day. She eats healthy foods such as salads, potatoes, soups, and fresh fruit. Yet, because her caloric intake is so low, she isn't receiving enough protein and other vital nutrients. So, keep in mind, the twenty pounds she's about to lose won't be the same twenty pounds she gained. The twenty pounds she gained at camp was pure fat. Through strict dieting, she will lose some fat but she will also lose some muscle. When she completes her diet she may weigh 90 pounds again, but her percentage of fat will no longer be 18 percent: it now may be 24 percent. Let's compare her post-diet body composition with her body composition results from steps 1 and 2.

21.6 pounds of Rachel's weight are fat
68.4 pounds are lean body mass

In step 1, when Rachel weighed 90 pounds, she had less body fat and more muscle!

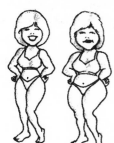

STEP 4: Because of the strict nature of her diet, Rachel begins to experience recurring bingeing episodes with some of her favorite foods that have been omitted from her diet. She begins to sneak food into her room and eat when no one is around. She now gains back the twenty pounds she lost. No muscle is added, only fat, so Rachel becomes even fatter.

Rachel becomes alarmed with the regained weight and tries even harder to stay on track and avoid junk food. Now, under her parents' watchful eye, the pressure is on her to do better. Still, the same thing keeps happening; she keeps gaining. When she weighs 110 pounds again, her percentage of fat has climbed to 37.8 percent. Here's her new body composition:

41.6 pounds of Rachel's weight are fat
68.4 pounds are lean body mass

STEP 5: The chart shows that Rachel is gaining more fat with each successive diet. As you can see from the body composition below, after another weight loss and weight gain cycle she's at her highest percentage of body fat despite several years of dieting. Naturally, her weight should increase as she gets older; however, for the sake of this example, I kept the weight constant so you could see what yo-yo dieting is really doing to her weight over the long term.

36 pounds of Rachel's weight are fat
54 pounds are lean body mass

In addition to the physical damage that dieting has done to her body, the emotional problems that she now has with food begin to manifest as well.

The concept here is simple: Put your child on a diet and you will destroy your child's chances of ever again having a healthy relationship with food. Besides ruining your child's relationship with food, dieting will change your child's metabolism, body composition, and attitudes about food. As a parent, you get blamed for enough things by your kids. Do you really need this, too?

Calorie Counting

It is important to educate your child on the concept of calories, but you don't want to create a constant calorie counter. Teach your child which foods generally contain more fat and calories than other alternatives. For example, your son is likely to understand that frozen yogurt is better for him than high fat ice cream. You need to teach him that lower calorie foods are good but you shouldn't teach him that starving is the answer.

While it is true that you have to shave back calories to a certain degree to lose weight, cutting them back too sharply causes additional problems. When calories are cut back drastically to lose weight, a child (like an adult) will experience hunger and deprivation. Once hunger sets in, even the thickest steel locks won't stop your son from sneaking food the first chance he gets. Control vanishes and bingeing begins. Because most children do not have free rein in the pantry, what is a boy or girl to do when hunger sets in and a parent is restricting what he or she eats?

As already mentioned, a harsh calorie-restricted diet often results in muscle loss, affecting a child's growth. His body will dip into its muscle to provide the fuel needed for him to walk, talk, and play during the day. The muscles will provide the vitamins, minerals, amino acids, and water that the diet does not. In other words, your child's body decides that muscle is expendable and fat is not. This is not good!

When muscle is gained, the metabolic rate speeds up and more calories are burned. When muscle is being lost, the metabolic rate slows down and fewer calories are burned. Therefore, to effectively help your child lose weight, you want him to maintain his muscle so that his metabolic rate remains high. Exercise and eating correctly will increase a child's muscle mass and metabolic rate. Dieting can cause serious problems down the road for your child in the form of a slower metabolism and difficulties with eating normal amounts of food and maintaining proper body weight. Calorie restrictions early in life can lead to permanent misconceptions and preoccupations with food.

Why does our metabolic rate slow down when we cut calories below a certain level? This is a perplexing question, but the answer I prefer, and which seems logical to me, is that it is probable that humans evolved under the constant threat of famine. Consequently, our bodies learned to respond to a reduction in calories and that response served as a natural defense mechanism against starvation. When the body is deprived of food for a certain length of time, it adjusts itself, by lowering the metabolic rate, in order to conserve its diminished nutrients and calories.

Unfortunately, the body cannot tell the difference between being lost on a desert island and starving, or sitting in a chair at home and purposely withholding food. It can only judge the circumstances based on how much and how frequently we eat. After a few weeks of strict dieting, the body goes into a sort of protective alert. In order to prevent starvation, the basal metabolic rate, the rate at which the body burns calories when at rest, begins to decline. In addition, the body uses muscle as fuel in an effort to preserve fat.

Both of these changes result in the body burning fewer and fewer calories, thereby making it more and more difficult to lose weight.

Several years of yo-yo dieting will make it difficult for a child—or an adult—to reach a reasonable body weight. His weight continues to climb as the years pass. By the time you consult a professional, he may have developed a distorted viewpoint concerning food, body image, and dieting.

Dieting Leads to Roadblocks

Here are examples of roadblocks that occur when a child is placed on a diet.

The First Roadblock
Remember how everything that Rachel did to lose weight was self-defeating? Because she lost so much muscle, her metabolic rate slowed down. Now, after repeated dieting, if she consumed the same number of calories she used to when she was at a normal weight, she would still gain several pounds every year just by eating a normal amount of food.

The Second Roadblock
The second problem is the appearance of Rachel's body. Each time she reached her goal weight, she had acquired more body fat than the time before. So she still may not fit into her clothes properly. Through poor dieting techniques, her body composition changed so much over the years that she does not like her reflection in the mirror. As your child ages, even if she is able to maintain her goal weight, she continues to tell herself that she needs to lose more weight just to look the same as she did before she began dieting. Thus, the diet process becomes a vicious cycle.

The Third Roadblock
Bingeing episodes continue even after Rachel has regained her weight. Mentally, the cravings for sweets and other foods continue for months to come. Since she is unable to control the intense cravings and bingeing, her weight is destined to fluctuate. These problems are a direct result of the self-imposed starvation, rigid deprivation, and harsh guidelines. Destined to repeat another dieting episode similar to the ones described, Rachel ends up complicating the weight problem by her psychological problems with food.

The Fourth Roadblock
One dangerous consequence of dieting may be that your child decides that the only way to control her weight is by not eating at all, so she slowly begins exerting too much

control over her food. As time progresses, she becomes obsessed with exercise. You see her losing weight and reward her with compliments; therefore, she forges ahead with determination. Soon, you notice that she is getting a little too thin and finally realize that she doesn't really eat anymore. You now realize she is exhibiting anorexic tendencies. Now a lifetime of new struggles with food begins.

The Fifth Roadblock

Maybe your child appears perfectly normal to everyone. She has lost weight, appears to be keeping it off, and eats a balanced diet. But unknown to you, friends, or family, she is harboring a deep, dark secret—bulimia. She eats normally for a few days or weeks, then suddenly, she binges on excessive amounts of food and then throws up to purge herself of the excess fat and calories. And believe it or not, her bulimic tendencies all started because of your attempt to help.

Still More Problems

Another aspect of dieting may take place in your daughter's saga of weight loss: She may have adopted a defeatist attitude because each time her dieting attempts have met with failure. As time passed, negative self-expectancies developed and she learned that any attempt at weight loss was a waste of time. Consequently, she gave up completely, admitted defeat, and resolved herself to a lifetime of obesity.

Measures of Progress

If weighing your child, counting calories or dieting are not good ways to evaluate the success of a weight control program, how can you tell whether your child is making any progress? Overall, your focus should be on supervising your children so they eat better and get more exercise, not on how much they weigh. Perhaps the best way to determine whether your daughter is making progress is by her appearance and how her clothes fit. It really doesn't matter how much she weighs, as long as she appears healthy and fits in regular-size clothes. Take into consideration that some kids are naturally bigger than others. Also, a child's weight isn't supposed to stay the same. Your son's growing body, increased muscle size and bone density will sometimes cause his weight on the bathroom scale to rise even as he drops body fat.

Five Ways to Measure Your Child's Progress

Here are five procedures by which to measure your child's progress; note that they avoid the daily ritual of stepping onto the scale.

1. *Body composition.* A body composition test determines what percentage of a person's weight is fat and what percentage is muscle, bone and other lean tissue. This test can also indicate the rate at which your child's body is developing. There

are about thirty different methods for determining body composition and each can yield a different result. A doctor, nutritionist, or other professional may perform a body composition test every four to six months. Because a body composition calculation yields a relative measurement from one time to the next, be certain to stick with the same technician and the same formula to ensure valid comparative results. A body composition measurement that indicates decreasing fat shows progress.

2. *Positive food selections.* If your daughter is making more positive food selections, she is doing better even if those selections fall short of being perfect. The goal is progress, not perfection. If she wants to eat a high fat food she hasn't had for a while, let her. Remember, occasional bad choices are part of healthy eating habits.

3. *Less guilt.* In the same vein, if your daughter feels less guilt about eating so-called forbidden foods, she's doing better. Progress is being made. Encourage her as she learns to manage her favorite foods rather than avoid them.

4. *Incorporation of regular exercise.* Is a regular activity or sport now part of your child's routine? Regular exercise is one of the best indicators of long-term success for losing and maintaining weight.

5. *Maintenance of weight.* As you will see in the following chapter, I do not advocate the weight scale as a measure except in very limited circumstances, such as gauging maintenance of weight during a time your son might normally gain. If he gains only two pounds during the holiday season rather than his usual ten, he is making positive strides. Like all journeys, the road to better health and weight control has bumps, yellow caution lights, stop signs, and detours. Reassure your child that there will be times when it just isn't possible to lose weight, and that's okay.

Chapter 3

The Psychology of Deprivation

What Is a Healthy Relationship with Food?

A healthy relationship with food begins in childhood. It is the ability to be around food without the constant urge to eat. It's understanding that the bag of potato chips or cookies in the pantry won't disappear if you don't eat them right away. For a nation of consumers who have been trained by advertisers that immediate gratification is the reward for personal success, the whole concept of food responsibility is contrary to the constant messages of uncontrolled abundance that bombard our senses. A healthy relationship with food certainly does mean that you can treat yourself to short vacations (eating bad foods) from sensible eating occasionally and not feel any guilt. A child in control of her relationship with food should not be preoccupied with food or talk about it all the time. Is your child in control of food or does food control your child? If the latter is true, your child does *not* have a healthy relationship with food.

What Causes an Unhealthy Relationship with Food?

The main factor that leads to problems with food is deprivation. If you put your son on a diet and tell him he cannot have his favorite foods, he will perceive the deprivation as a form of punishment. His own benefit notwithstanding, he, like other children, will consider food control as punishment.

Once a child has been deprived of food, there seems to be a change in his focus pertaining to it. At first, food avoidance may be easy, but eventually, thoughts about certain foods intensify. We know that a restricted diet causes changes in brain chemistry, with the result that when the child is allowed to eat again normally, he consumes food to an extreme. The desire to gorge may persist for weeks or months. As the loss of control becomes apparent, the concerned parent may try to force her child to diet again, but each regimen is shorter and the child repeats the bingeing cycle.

It seems that with children the more frequently food is withheld, the more powerful is the loss of their control.

Of course, there are other factors that affect a child's eating behavior. The size of a family can play a role. For example, a child with many brothers and sisters learns early to compete with her siblings for food. It doesn't stay in the house very long; snacks disappear within a day or two after Mom does the shopping.

Sometimes an unhealthy relationship with food develops because it has been used as a replacement for love and as a reward. No doubt about it, food does make us feel better. But if it is used as a pacifier to soothe us during childhood, or to smooth over problems, the children will rely on it in the same fashion when they grow up.

Another contributor to a child's unhealthy relationship with food is teasing or taunting by other children, siblings, or parents. One day, I came home crying from school because I had decided my ears were too big. Some of the kids had nicknamed me Dumbo. I had never before thought my ears looked different, but once I was tagged, other kids started teasing me as well. Although the teasing didn't last, I became overly sensitive about my ears. I was convinced that people stared at my ears. My dad tried to soothe me, but to no avail. Eventually, he took me to see a plastic surgeon. The surgeon explained my two options: (1) allow him to cut the muscles located at the back of my ears so that they would lay back and no longer stick out; or (2) understand that my ears had grown faster than the rest of me and I would grow into them within a year or two. I chose the second option. Yes, I did grow into my ears. Time truly is a great healer. By understanding that my ears had outpaced the rest of me, and that I could make the final decision about surgery, I felt in control again.

For an overweight child who is teased and taunted, time may not heal the scars, because she feels trapped in her body. The first and most devastating remarks that children hear about their bodies often come from within their own household, not from the school yard. Kids who are mercilessly teased can become depressed or act out their frustration by becoming mean or withdrawn. A brother who constantly calls his sister "fatso" contributes to her misery out of proportion to the size of the insult. In extreme cases, an overweight child may internalize such criticism to the point that it becomes the lever for her withdrawal from social activities, or she might have difficulty establishing lasting relationships.

The Psychology of Deprivation

As I stated early in this chapter, food deprivation has a discernible cycle. It is worth reviewing briefly. You and your daughter decide she needs to lose weight. The first thing you do is place limits on her snacking and remove all bad foods. For the first two weeks, she does really well. You consistently compliment her, tell her how proud you are, and continue to offer support. Then, like a bolt of lightning, she gets struck down by cravings. These cravings strike from all directions: television, radio, even the ice cream truck ringing its bell two blocks away. After a short time, your daughter gives in to the urge to eat and finally binges on a forbidden food. After the binge, she feels remorse, intensified by the fact that she violated your rules. Next, she begins to rationalize and justify her behavior. Her internal voice says, "Well, since I've already blown it, I might as well really blow it."

Don't Slit the Other Three Tires

It's important to teach your child not to lose perspective over a momentary bump in the road. Bad choices are a part of healthy, normal eating. It's the rigid, harsh and deprived styles of eating that lead to unhealthy relationships with food. Because bad choices are a part of healthy eating, it's up to you to teach your child how to incorporate the occasional bad choice into an overall, lifelong plan of healthy eating. Dieters tend to become overly involved with mistakes, which only makes matters worse. When a bad day of eating occurs, it doesn't signify total failure.

Think of a bad food decision in terms of a flat tire on your car. If you are driving down the road on an extended journey (toward healthier eating, perhaps) and your car has a flat tire (a bad food choice), do you jump out of the car and slit the other three tires? Of course not! More likely, you would put on the spare and continue on your way, grateful that the other three tires didn't go flat.

Part of our strategy involves making Better Bad Choices, which we will discuss at length in the following chapter. If your car has one of those dinky spare tires that resemble an oversized donut, you can begin to grasp the concept of Better Bad Choices. Everyone would agree that a compact spare is not as desirable to drive on as a full-size tire, but given the above circumstances, it is a better option than a blown-out full-size tire, and it allows you to keep moving forward on your journey toward better, healthier eating. Flat tires will occur, but they don't have to result in a binge that, in effect, slashes the other three tires on the car.

Birth of a Binge

If Your Child is Bingeing

A binge doesn't just happen or strike randomly. In most cases, bingeing is actually a step-by-step process your child goes through. By understanding the evolution of thoughts behind the binge, you will be better prepared to help your child overcome the common feelings of guilt that accompany bingeing.

A binge almost always begins with a catalyst of some sort. In most cases it's a negative feeling or emotion that triggers the desire to eat and feel comforted. On any given day, a child encounters all kinds of negative situations. Some days these feelings trigger a binge; other days they don't. The intensity of her feelings depends on how your daughter is interpreting the world around her on a particular day. Some triggers may not affect her if everything else is going well; yet the same trigger on a bad day may evoke an intense desire to eat.

Anger, boredom, anxiety over an upcoming spelling test, or a problem with a friend are common triggers. Often too young to understand the source of uncomfortable feelings, a child may be unable to cope with her troubling thoughts. Instead, she turns to food to make herself feel better. Food and feeling better are a natural association for a child. After all, when we stick a bottle in a baby's mouth the empty feeling of hunger goes away. But we must help our children recognize that food is not an effective way to cope with life's problems.

In some cases, the food trigger may not be associated with a negative emotional state at all. Hunger alone can act as a catalyst to binge. Maybe your daughter is skipping breakfast or not eating enough nutritious snacks and becomes victim of a legitimate craving for food. The bottom line is that the stimulus to binge happens for a lot of different reasons. Whether it's disappointment over a bad report card or a broken toy, or a craving that results from improper eating, be aware that your child may be frustrated and is trying to cure it with food.

If you understand the cycle of bingeing, you will be able to identify the action signals in your child's behavior. Help her deal with her frustration, rather than creating a bigger problem by giving her food to make her feel better.

It's Followed by a Decision and Action

Once the bingeing catalyst is triggered, your child will make a conscious decision to eat something. This decision has two parts. On the one hand, the decision to eat is manifested when your son simply reaches for food or asks you for it first. Second, he may delay his binge until later when no one else can observe him. A child may spend hours planning the binge. He may slip out to a local store and purchase a large quantity of candy, hiding it until he is alone, and then eat everything at one time. When your son finally gives in to the urge to eat, he will consume much more than normal to make up for the long hours of intense deprivation.

As I described earlier, after the binge, your son engages in a typical thought process: "I've already binged, so I might as well eat everything else I can get my hands on because I know I will have to start my diet again tomorrow. If Mom and Dad knew what I did, they would be so mad at me."

Now Comes the Guilt

After a child binges, he may feel a sense of shame, remorse, and hopelessness. Perhaps he feels as if he has misbehaved. Now he may experience a feeling of shame and reduced self-esteem, which can act as a trigger for bingeing all over again. Bingeing has nothing to do with a lack of will power. It stems from feelings of deprivation and stress. Keep in mind that your son is probably oblivious to the stimulus that caused his binge eating and takes himself to task for being weak, which adds to his depression and low self-esteem. If he had been following the right kind of eating program, his downward spiral could have been prevented.

The Morning-After Blues

As the feelings of guilt set in, your son may feel melancholy and blue. These feelings may have one or more of the following characteristics:

A. *Immediate reaction.* He may feel guilty immediately, as soon as he finishes eating the forbidden food. Immediate guilt, in turn, causes more stress and the desire to eat begins to build all over again.

B. *Delayed reaction.* Have you ever eaten your way through the holidays, only to look in the mirror on January 2 and say to yourself, "What on earth have I done?" Your child might be tempted to let down his guard "just while I'm at camp," or "while I'm at Grandma's house; after all, I'm on vacation." Later, when he reflects on his actions, even if all he did was eat what everyone else was eating, he may become overwhelmed with guilt.

C. *Emotional reaction.* Guilt, hopelessness, and helplessness are emotional hangovers that may accompany the blues. This is particularly true of a teenager who feels so out of control with her eating that food constantly seems to win. Classic examples are those of the bulimic or compulsive overeater.

D. *Physical reaction.* Your child may feel ill from the quantity of food he has eaten, ranging from feeling bloated, to nauseated, to just plain sick.

NOTE: If I have been redundant in this chapter by reasserting earlier statements about the deprivation cycle, it is because this typical behavior underlies the major problem of on-and-off dieting. Unless we understand the cycle and the symptoms, and learn how to forestall them, we will never be able to guide our children into a weight control program that works.

The Spiral of Broken Promises

The child has arrived at this stage, with feelings of guilt, following a binge. It is not uncommon for her to promise herself never to binge again. With nothing but good intentions, she makes a personal vow to change and resolves to restart her diet "on Monday."

When Monday comes, however, a disappointment at school—a poor grade on a spelling test—can lead to another bad choice—a frosted brownie or a Kit Kat bar. She may rationalize a single bad choice, but later in the week she finds it easier to decide to have pizza with the astronomy club and ice cream with the kids in band. By the end of the week, it becomes apparent that she hasn't resumed her diet. Eventually, she begins to doubt that she is capable of keeping her promises to herself and ultimately stops believing she will ever lose her unwanted weight.

The result of her broken promises is a spiraling pattern of self-defeating thoughts. Each time that she promises herself to "do better" and then stumbles, she realizes she is lying to herself. The more she lies, the less she believes in herself. As time goes on, her self-doubt builds to such a point that it overrides any attempt to change. Before long, she binges every time she encounters certain emotional triggers.

All of our future expectations are based upon past experiences. A child may decide at an early age that he is not successful because he has failed each time he has tried. If a child's experience is checkered with failures, is it surprising that he develops a negative self-expectation? Along with the failures come negative feelings such as humiliation, low self-esteem, ridicule, and myriad other undesirable emotions. It is only natural that a wall is built that prevents him from trying again. And is it surprising that the mantle of failure, with which he has cloaked himself in respect to weight control, spreads to include all of his ambitions?

Breaking the Binge Cycle

How do we break the binge cycle? First and foremost, we must recognize that deprivation is at the root of most bingeing behavior. That's why it's important never to place a child on a strict diet that prevents him from eating all of his favorite foods. Cutting out all junk food may *sound* like a good idea, but the result will be a child who sneaks out to eat whenever possible. Before long, you will be discovering empty pizza boxes and candy wrappers hidden under his bed. When the evidence accumulates that bingeing seems to be your son's major response to his life's daily stresses, there are three keys with which you can help him break the binge cycle:

1. *First, to intercept the binge, identify the catalyst.* Identify the catalyst that triggers your son's bingeing episodes and then teach him how to implement new coping skills and strategies. If boredom is a catalyst, get your son involved in a new hobby or sport. Perhaps he could volunteer a little time by tutoring a younger student. Are there any interesting clubs at his school or in your neighborhood? Try to reduce your child's stress and teach him how to control negative emotions in a more positive way.

   Communicate with your son to find out what is going on in his world—"Are you still upset with Hunter? He is your best friend." "Are you worried about that math test on Thursday?" Your job is to sit down with your son or daughter and communicate that you are ready to help. And you must convince him or her that your offer is genuine and it is not motivated by a parental desire to control or interfere. Also remember, a kid who doesn't share his feelings may have pent-up negative emotions that manifest in other ways. For example, an angry child may be mean to other kids or pout about seemingly meaningless situations.

A good parent is a lot like a good detective. It's difficult for kids to articulate why they behave the way they do, so you must study the clues and draw your own conclusions.

2. *Help your child make Better Bad Choices.* Even if you cannot convert your child to truly healthy foods, you can make progress by always having Better Bad Choices available to her. By using the Better Bad Choice concept, your kids can eat foods they enjoy without excess calories and guilt.

3. *Have alternatives ready at the point of decision.* Remove your child from high-risk situations that trigger the desire to eat. Offer fruit rather than twelve kinds of cookies for a snack. If your son always wants a fast food taco after school, drive home by a different route to avoid the Taco Bell along the way.

Chapter 4

Better Bad Choices

Many people are largely defined by what they do for a living. For example, you may decide that cheating other people of money, or being late for work, is not a quality you wish to possess.So you show up for work on time, you stay late if necessary, and you are willing to give 110 percent to your job. We also define ourselves in spiritual ways. Maybe you are Christian or Jewish and thus you live within guidelines of your religion. You don't kill people, you don't lie, and you try your best to help your fellow man. You are also defined by your relationships. Maybe you and your spouse have decided how you want to handle arguments or have agreed what type of schools you want your kids to attend, but have you ever spent time defining yourself as a healthy person? It's time to think about how you and your family will live your lives as healthy people, because once you give thought to this area of your life, you instantly set down parameters or guidelines by which to live. Maybe you decide to give up red meat or fried foods. Maybe you switch from whole milk to skim. Whatever the changes are, you need to begin on them today by asking yourself how you want to see you family living a healthy lifestyle.

Throughout this book, as you've noticed, I use the term "Better Bad Choices." I have waited until now to define it clearly, because I am sure you have already reached your own conclusion as to the meaning.

By Better Bad Choices, I mean the selection of foods to fit into a weight control program that are better than the worst choices. In other words, two cups of low fat ice cream is a better choice than two cups of high fat ice cream for the same portion. The difference in calories is staggering. Two cups of regular premium high fat ice cream contain 1120 calories, while an equal size serving of low fat ice cream contains only 400 calories.

This chapter is devoted to explaining Better Bad Choices. I think you will be surprised at the variety of tasty, appealing low fat alternatives that fit into an effective lifetime weight control program.

Now, everyone knows that proper diet and exercise is the only way to achieve and maintain optimum weight and health. We've examined why traditional dieting does more harm than good, because "diets" are always based on some form of deprivation, which exacerbates the problems of overweight eaters.

We've also established the importance of building a successful program of healthy eating and weight control for our children, and ourselves, on a positive foundation of support and unconditional love. The best way to begin building is by avoiding the "dieter's mentality," and thereby avoiding deprivation. Instead, we must develop a new way of thinking when it comes to food. Abolish the idea that your child cannot eat any bad foods, and get ready to adopt a new way of introducing your child's favorite foods.

Start with Better Bad Choices

Helping your child develop healthy eating habits isn't difficult. It merely requires serving the right foods the majority of the time, while serving the wrong foods only occasionally. During my early years as a nutritionist, long before the wave of fat-free products became the rage, I developed a unique approach to help children satisfy cravings without giving up their favorite foods. That was when I came up with the title Better Bad Choices, and this concept has become the cornerstone of my program. The goal is to help your child "do better" with food choices, not take them away. I wanted parents and children to know that bad choices are a part of normal eating and that attempting to eat perfectly only creates strong preoccupations with food, leading to failure. (Remember the anatomy of a binge?)

Better Bad Choices are not synonymous with bad choices, as I pointed out at the beginning of this chapter. Let me explain further. No one would say that a soft drink containing 70 empty calories from sugar and no other nutritional value is a good choice, but compared to a regular cola—with its jolt of caffeine and 170 empty calories from sugar—the 70 calorie option is certainly a Better Bad Choice, especially if it satisfies your son's craving for a sweet drink.

Likewise, a lower fat snack cracker, which may contain a higher percentage of fat than we would otherwise recommend, is still a Better Bad Choice than a high fat potato chip. Lower fat foods usually contain fewer calories than higher fat choices. If your daughter simply chooses a lower fat alternative of the same type of food, often she can satisfy her craving while still dropping body fat.

Incorporating Better Bad Choices is a realistic and effective strategy for progressively healthier eating and weight control. Better Bad Choices are not an admission of defeat; they are a practical option for eating in the real world. If, by utilizing Better Bad Choices, your daughter gains control of her eating decisions, over time she will feel empowered to make increasingly better choices.

There are three ways to utilize the Better Bad Choice approach.

1. *Help your child make more positive food selections.* By making more positive food selections, you can remove a lot of fat and calories from your son's diet, yet still allow him to satisfy the craving and eat like a normal person. For example, instead of letting him eat regular potato chips, switch to pretzels. Serve baked foods rather than fried foods. Switch to diet Coke from regular Coke. Get the picture?

    The most important place to start making Better Bad Choices is with your own cooking. Your family will immediately reap the benefits of better eating habits if you simply make lower fat substitutions for higher fat foods in your diet. By using chicken broth or cooking spray in your sauté pan instead of oil, for example, the amount of fat and calories added to your meal can be substantially reduced. Through use of properly seasoned ground turkey breast instead of ground beef, skim milk instead of whole milk, and lite ice cream instead of premium ice cream, your family can enjoy an endless array of healthy foods without all the fat and calories.

2. *Reduce the frequency of bad eating.* If your family normally eats high fat Mexican food three times a week, change your habits to only have Mexican food once every ten days or so. By reducing the frequency of eating high fat foods, your daughter can significantly reduce her overall calorie and fat intake. Simply trading baked chips for fried chips and cutting out the cheese in one Mexican food meal can save hundreds of calories and over fifty grams of fat, which inevitably will translate into a loss of body fat over time!

3. *Reduce the amount of food your child eats.* If your son usually eats a whole pizza, and now is only eating half, this is a Better Bad Choice. The same goes for eating half a basket of chips at the Mexican restaurant instead of a whole basket.

Of course, the best way to improve your child's diet is to implement a combination of all three approaches. Instead of giving your daughter a twelve ounce T-bone steak five times a week, serve her a six ounce, extra-lean sirloin steak once a week.

I know these ideas sound overly simple and, perhaps, obvious; but trust me, they work. And it should help you to know that your daughter doesn't have to be rigid and perfect with her diet in order to make significant progress.

Today, more than ever, companies are scrambling to create as many fat-free foods as possible. They know that descriptions such as "reduced fat," "fat-free," and "light" sell foods. With all the fat-free foods now readily available, already you may be making Better Bad Choices for your children. My purpose here is to urge you to continue more deliberately and consistently to use the Better Bad Choices approach.

Better Bad Choices make it possible for you to guide your child easily into healthier eating habits. Better Bad Choices confront the problem head on and provide a bridge for your child to gain control over his eating and his weight.

Once you master the concept of Better Bad Choices, you will realize that there is nothing your child cannot eat. It simply requires substituting lower fat alternatives for higher fat foods when preparing recipes, and choosing lower fat and lower calorie alternatives when you go out to eat. The longer you continue to focus on Better Bad Choices for the whole family, the progression to healthy eating becomes easier and easier. Focusing on Better Bad Choices takes the emphasis off of your child's weight and places it where it should be—on better overall eating habits and exercise. Gaining mastery involves having a shopping list and a menu planning strategy that incorporates Better Bad Choices. We will tackle these important elements in chapter 5.

Be Careful: Fat-Free Doesn't Mean No Calories

There are pitfalls along the Better Bad Choices pathway. With so many Better Bad Choices available, why do we continue to get fatter? Unfortunately, many fat-free products contain almost the same number of calories as the regular foods! Try this: compare reduced fat chocolate chip cookies to regular. You will be surprised to find that the reduced fat variety actually has more calories! If your daughter eats an entire bag of regular Chips Ahoy at 50 calories per cookie, she will ingest 1,700 calories. But if she eats the same amount of SnackWell chocolate chip cookies, she will ingest 2,040 calories! Similarly, fat-free chips have 110 calories an ounce; an ounce is only about ten chips.

If you let your son eat bigger portions of fat-free foods than he would eat of unreduced fat foods, believing he will lose weight, think again. Even low fat foods can add extra calories. When you help your child to make Better Bad Choices, you must take into consideration total calories as well as fat content.

Establishing a Healthy Relationship with Food

In addition to the three-pronged approach to implementing Better Bad Choices, the following steps and guidelines will help your child establish a healthy relationship with food.

Never Place Your Child on a Diet

I have already emphasized the perils of dieting, but it is worthwhile here to reiterate some weight control facts that you may use as a guide to help your child. Kids should never be judged by how much weight they lose or fail to lose. The focus should be on developing and managing a healthy lifetime eating plan. Let's take the focus off his weight and place the emphasis where it really counts, on being more active and eating better. I can't stress this point enough: *Dieting leads to nothing but problems.*

Implement Small Frequent Meals and Snacks

The only way your child will feel in control over food is if he doesn't experience hunger. Frequent meals, coupled with nutritious nibbling, will keep him from getting hungry. As I outline later in this chapter, a child's eating plan should be set up around breakfast, lunch, and dinner, but also should include a midafternoon mini-meal, and if possible, a midmorning snack. Frequent meals are the most important tool to increase a child's metabolism, prevent hunger, and supply more energy.

All cravings begin with a single thought that originates in one of several ways. *Thinking* about a certain food may stimulate the craving. *Smelling* a food stimulates the image that drives the craving. *Seeing* a particular food can certainly generate the thought that creates the craving. In each case, the thought precedes the craving. Hunger intensifies the need to find food. If you make sure that your son eats frequent, healthy meals and well-balanced snacks, then you will almost guarantee that his thoughts about food won't be intense.

Nutritious Nibbling

Were you raised to believe that snacking between meals is bad? If your answer is yes, you need to reprogram your thinking. Throughout this book I've been stressing the concept that a child should never be deprived. Although the concept that you have to eat in order to lose may go against everything you ever heard about weight loss, it is the only certain method by which your son or daughter can develop a healthy relationship with food. Although having a midmorning snack during school may not be possible for your daughter, you can give her a midmorning snack on weekends.

Never Make Your Child Clean Her Plate

While you were growing up were you told that you should clean your plate because of all the starving kids in China? I can't count the times I fervently wished that the food on my plate could be sent over there to help those poor kids. Don't force your daughter to continue eating when she is full. That is a form of force feeding, and after she has made a habit of eating more than she wants, she may find it difficult to ever leave food on her plate. Also, don't ever offer your child a reward for finishing the food on her plate. Making a promise like, "I'll give you some ice cream for dessert if you finish your food," only makes matters worse. If she is already full from the clean plate rule, and then you promise dessert if she will exceed her capacity, what do you think will start to happen? No great mystery. She'll soon join the legion of overweight kids.

Let Your Child Choose How Much Food to Eat at Mealtimes

You are in control of what foods your child eats simply by purchasing healthy foods and Better Bad Choices. But a child should always control how much food she eats at meals. Don't ever cut your daughter off at mealtime. Let her appetite dictate when she is full. Center the table talk around healthy conversations about school activities, sports, or other interests. But never discuss her eating habits at the dinner table unless she brings up the subject.

Let Your Child Do What Comes Naturally

Certainly you don't want your kids coloring the walls with lipstick, but there are more productive things that come to children naturally. They like to be in perpetual motion: running, climbing, playing. Encourage your son to play and enjoy himself but try to avoid making him grow up too soon by assuming adult roles. Restrictive eating isn't natural. Let your child grow into his weight by becoming more active and by reducing fat and calorie intake.

Seek the Help of a Professional

Don't be reluctant to consult a nutritionist, therapist, or other professional if you don't know the best way to help your daughter lose weight or increase self-esteem. Sometimes you just can't fix the problem on your own. Many times it's better to engage a neutral person as the one suggesting treatment options.

Cook More at Home

Because many kids come home to an empty house after school, it's easy to understand why they consume a lot of junk food. They reach for fast, easy foods like sodas, chips, and candy bars until you arrive home. By the time you roll in, exhausted, it may not matter what you decide to cook for dinner, because they're already full from snacking. If the meal you cook goes uneaten, you may decide that eating out is easier. Sure it is, but unfortunately, "easier" often means relying on more fast food, pizza, and cafeterias.

It's a fact: A stressed-out family life overrides healthy eating habits. But you must bring order to mealtimes if you really want to improve your child's eating, as well as the rest of the family's. You can still eat out twice a week but try cooking at home more often. Eating out actually takes more time and usually causes more stress. Consider how much time is spent getting the kids ready, driving to the restaurant, ordering, eating, and driving back home. It's at least an hour-long ordeal.

Eating at home can and should be a positive experience—not rushed.

Parents should enlist the support of their children in this endeavor. By participating in home meals, the children learn responsibility and are involved in the cooking preparation, where important skills are taught. Family participation at the table increases the child's sense of belonging as well as the lesson that more relaxed dining at home is more fun and less stressful than running out to a restaurant every time hunger sets in. And one of the bonuses of cooking at home is that there are leftovers for the following day's lunches.

What about Eating Out?

McDonald's is usually the first restaurant a child goes to. Believe it or not, almost all children recognize Ronald McDonald by the age of two years. Among children it's the number one requested place to eat. That's no surprise, but did you know that one order of Chicken McNuggets, a small order of fries, and a Coke contain 690 calories and 33 grams of fat? The soda alone contains about ten teaspoons of sugar!

Try to reduce the frequency of your family's visits to restaurants. Children tend to consume twice as many calories when they eat out, in part because restaurant food contains hidden fat and calories. When you prepare meals at home, you are able to maintain control over the fat, salt, sugar, and calories your child consumes. Today, with all the single parents, dual working parents and late-working parents to account for, it's understandable why many families eat out more. If you must eat out, order wisely. You can ask the waiter to remove fat by requesting no skin on the chicken, no butter on the vegetables or roll, and salad dressing on the side. And, as I have touched on before, it's vital to establish regular eating times for your child. Preferably, the whole family can sit down together, not only to eat, but to discover and discuss what is going on with individual family members. Open family communication alleviates the daily stress and pressures that often are responsible for overeating.

The appendix to this book contains a section with the caloric and fat values for menu items from most popular fast food establishments. This list will enable you and your child to select Better Bad Choices whenever the family has to eat out at one of these places.

Cook Food that Satisfies Your Child

Here is a common scenario: Your kid has been following a diet for the last several weeks. Things seem to be going great. Then all of a sudden one day, like a bolt of lightning, the cravings strike. Wham! Without any forewarning, your son is unable to control the urge to eat a bag of Fritos. To make matters worse, it doesn't stop there. Next, you find empty pizza boxes under his bed and a stack of candy wrappers under the pile of old newspapers in the trash can.

Once the urge to eat begins to settle down, your son feels a sense of guilt. You realize this when it occurs to you that he hasn't looked you in the eye for three days. Ultimately, he begins to belittle himself and wonder why he lacks the will power to eat right for more than a few weeks at a time. For a person who fails to follow a rigid program, the reason has less to do with a personal weakness than with a lack of understanding of the human need to be satisfied by the foods we eat.

I've discussed this before, as well as the subject of deprivation, but there is another aspect to deprivation that you should understand. When we think of deprivation, the first thing that comes to mind usually is a lack of food or a calorie deficiency. In most cases, however, the actual source of deprivation stems from poor cooking skills or habits. Most dieters have been conditioned to think of dieting as eating very bland foods. "Eating healthy" used to mean opening a can of water-packed tuna and forking it right out of the can with plain rice as a complement. An alternative was a grilled plain chicken breast with a dry baked potato.

Although a healthy diet will include basic foods such as chicken, rice, and baked potatoes, how these foods are prepared makes all the difference.

Why Food Should Taste Great

To feel satisfied from a meal, it takes a combination of flavors, textures, colors, and moisture. Satiety—feeling satisfied—requires all of these factors. We have three different kinds of taste buds that respond to sweet, salty, and bitter substances, and cravings for all these tastes need to be satisfied. In most cases dieters eat foods that lack one or more of these important characteristics. For example, a plain grilled chicken breast has one flavor and one texture. That's it. The same goes for dry rice, plain grilled fish, and water packed tuna. Don't get me wrong! Your child may actually enjoy plain grilled chicken; but after eating the same flavor and texture day after day, she could eat thirty pounds of chicken and feel full but still unsatisfied. Two bland flavors and two textures are not enough to satisfy anyone for very long.

Have you ever opened your cooler of food at work, looked inside, shut the lid, and headed out for Mexican food? Have you ever thought, "If I see another piece of chicken, I will grow feathers and fly right out the window?" You and your child do not have to settle for a bland and boring diet. To prove it, I've included delicious, simple to prepare recipes in the back of the book, which achieve our goals of great taste, variety, and reduced fat.

Pack Great Tasting Lunches!

Make sure that the foods you pack in your daughter's lunchbox taste great. Get in the habit of experimenting with new foods. Let's face it: If you pack boring, bland food, it's only a matter of time before your daughter will search for more interesting food at school—chips, fries, ice cream, or candy. Make sure that you add variety. Try a new food each week and see what appeals to her.

You Have to Be Creative

It requires ingenuity on your part to help your child successfully reach her long-term goal of healthy eating. But like anything else, cooking becomes a lot more fun once you get the hang of it. Take rice, for example. Most people simply boil water and rice together and consider it cooked. Not me. Instead of water, I use defatted chicken broth. After the rice is cooked, I toss in a handful of dried cranberries or cherries. Now, instead of having one flavor and one texture, I have several. The rice takes on a slightly yellow color from the chicken broth and has a touch of chicken aroma and flavor. The dried cranberries add a touch of burgundy and a slightly tart bite. My way of cooking rice didn't take any additional time. Which rice do you think your child would prefer?

Does your vision of a tuna salad sandwich for your child's lunch consist of a can of water packed tuna dumped in a bowl, mixed with fat-free mayonnaise, and then spread between slices of bread? Even though it may taste okay, it lacks the colors, textures, and additional flavors that create satiety. Try this: Before you mix the water packed tuna with the fat-free mayonnaise, toss in water chestnuts, dill relish, dill seasoning, diced celery and onion, and maybe a touch of garlic powder and pepper. Spread it on bread that has been toasted, along with lettuce and tomato. My sandwich won't take much longer than yours to prepare, but which do you think will taste more satisfying? It's these simple kinds of interesting tastes and textures that keep children eating correctly for a lifetime and loving what they eat. Naturally, your child's tastes may differ from mine, so it's important to use items *they* like (raisins, carrots, etc.).

Do You Eat the Same Meals Over and Over?

Studies have shown that the normal American eating pattern consists of fifteen meals. The average person chooses between two breakfasts (with an occasional third option), and rotates five different lunches and seven dinners. Think about this for a minute. Your daughter probably eats cereal or toast each morning, a sandwich or hot dog for lunch, and either meat, pasta, or a hamburger for dinner. Do you often go to the same restaurants and order the same things? It's human nature to eat within a circle of food choices and rarely venture outside those choices.

As you can see, it is important to develop at least fifteen recipes that you and your family like, but don't stop there. Develop as many low fat recipes as possible. Many recipes can be quickly modified by making a few switches. For example, if you have a chicken stir-fry that everyone loves, try substituting shrimp in place of the chicken breast. The added variety will enhance your enjoyment and avoid boredom with the same recipes. Different spices and assorted vegetables can creatively alter any recipe.

It seems that many dieters can only go about two weeks before deciding that donuts are the way to cure eating boredom. But before you agree, I'm going to share the reasons why I am rarely bored by the foods I eat. For starters, it's because I take the time to cook and prepare foods that taste great. So my mind rarely wanders to other food choices. Think about your own tastes for a minute. If you were going to eat grilled shrimp topped with a mango relish, a grilled Portabello mushroom with a grilled onion slice and sugar snap peas, wouldn't you look forward to eating? This meal is not complex; it's actually quite simple and takes less than fifteen minutes to prepare. And while I'm at it, I make extra for leftovers for lunch the next day.

Another reason I don't get bored is that I continually look for ways to implement variety. If I have grilled chicken breast for dinner one night, I'll simply place the leftover chicken in a food processor and add water chestnuts, celery, onions, mustard and dill seasoning. After processing all the ingredients together I end up with a really nice chicken salad for sandwiches. I'll place the salad on toast one day, and stuff it into a bell pepper the next.

The recipes in the back of this book will teach you how to cook simple but exciting foods that your children and the rest of the family will love. The recipes are designed to be fast, easy, and great tasting. Your mission, should you decide to accept it, is to try some new recipes and discover that you can offer your kids great foods that will help them lose weight without feeling deprived or bored! Entrees like Chicken Fingers, Turkey Burgers, and similar meals will have your kids asking for more.

Keith Klein's Top Ten Rules for Cooking Survival

1. Experiment and try new recipes. Take a little extra time to add colors and textures to each of your child's meals.
2. Modify high fat recipes that your child likes and convert them to lower fat versions by making substitutions. (See the substitution list in the recipes section.)
3. Shop at least once a week and try to find something new each time.
4. Double or triple the recipes so you will have leftovers for your child's lunch. Leftovers can be used in a variety of ways. For example, a turkey breast meatloaf makes a great meatloaf sandwich. Or a grilled chicken breast can be turned into a chicken salad sandwich.
5. Use condiments that don't add fat. Condiments add color and flavor that make foods look good and taste great.
6. To inject color and extra flavor, add vegetables that your child likes to every recipe. Because they are naturally low in fat and calories, vegetables may be eaten in unlimited quantities.
7. To prevent boredom, vary the foods your child eats every day .
8. Develop at least fifteen great tasting, easy-to-make recipes that your child likes.
9. To add moisture and flavor, marinate meats in low fat condiments before broiling or grilling.
10. Top plain grilled meats with low fat sauces to add flavor, taste, texture, moisture, and color.

Don't Override an Appetite

We all have a built-in appetite control center, which sends a signal to the brain when we're full and it's time to stop eating. It's important to eat slowly to give the brain a chance to tell us we're full before we overeat. Force feeding overrides a child's appetite control center. Forcing your son to eat everything on his plate is similar to force feeding. If this is done enough times, the body quits sending signals that it is full. If a child is forced to finish dinner and then eats dessert, a lot of damage can result. He will no longer be able to distinguish for himself when to quit eating, which inevitably leads to weight gain. Set a good example by eating slowly. It takes about thirty minutes for the bloodstream to send signals to the brain that you're full.

What do you do if your daughter wants dessert but didn't finish dinner? Let her know that dessert will be served when everyone else has finished eating. Let her clear the table or help with the dishes before serving dessert. Always serve dessert at least twenty minutes after the meal. By then, everyone's appetite will be diminished, which in turn reduces overall caloric intake. Serve Better Bad Choices for dessert and don't serve dessert after every dinner. A good dessert would be fresh fruit topped with a fat-free whipped cream. Also, make sure it's served and eaten at the table. In fact, all meals and snacks should be served at the table, never in front of the television.

Chapter 5

Get Ready, Get Set, Go!

School mornings at Rachel's house are hectic, to say the least. Dad leaves for work before Rachel even gets up. Mom works full-time too, yet she manages to get Rachel and her twin sister and brother off to school on time. They usually have a quick bowl of cereal and a banana before they leave, but Mom doesn't have time to pack their lunches.

At Blake's house, it's just Mom and him. Mom pushes the snooze button so many times that it's usually Blake who finally wakes her up. They rush around in the morning and rarely have time to sit down and share breakfast together. Blake usually eats toast in the car on the way to school. On a good day, mother and son may have time to stop and get an Egg McMuffin.

Rachel, the twins and Blake have a lot in common when it comes time for lunch. Each of them has been given money to buy lunch in the school cafeteria. At 11:30 each morning, they get to choose between pizza, fried chicken nuggets, a cheeseburger and fries, chips, ice cream, soda, or a healthy grilled chicken breast with steamed potatoes. It's not surprising that none of them can tell you if the chicken breast is good.

The path has been paved that these kids will follow into adulthood. Not only is morning a stressful time with limited, if any, time for breakfast, but lunch is not much better. They are likely to grow into adults who skip breakfast nine times out of ten and eat out for lunch every day. To make matters worse, when lunchtime finally arrives, their decisions are bound to be determined by what looks good and what is available, rather than by careful, healthy choices.

When I was a child, my mother always awakened the entire family early. She started breakfast while everyone got washed and dressed. My brother, sister, and I each had designated duties every morning: My sister set the table, my brother cleared it, and I washed the dishes. The best part was that the whole family sat down together and talked about the upcoming day. Later, when I was doing the dishes, my mom was busy getting ready for her job. When it was time to be dropped off at school, we all felt relaxed and calm. Mom made a lunch for us to take to school each day. And when we were old enough to make our own lunches, my mom taught us how, rather than letting us take our chances at the school cafeteria.

Mornings are still the most enjoyable time for me. As an adult, I still wake up early, but now I relish breakfast with my wife. And I still carry a lunch with me every day to work. My positive childhood experiences carried over into adulthood. But most important, I'm in control of my weight and my health.

How to Get Started

One of the first things you must do is to replace foods in your pantry that are too high in fat, calories, and salt. I have provided a suggested shopping list later in this chapter. You are the best judge of which foods will work for your family. Of course, buying alternative foods or Better Bad Choices is only one step; getting your children to actually taste them will depend a great deal on how you present them.

One evening, my nephew Shawn and I were at a local pizza parlor where we implemented a Better Bad Choice approach. We ordered a pizza with bell peppers, onions, and mushrooms, but no cheese. The missing cheese removed about six hundred fat calories. When Shawn first looked at the pizza, he exclaimed, "Hey, Uncle Keith, they forgot the cheese!" I know how much Shawn loves cheese. Here's how I handled it:

Keith: Shawn, have you ever eaten the crust of the pizza with a little tomato sauce still on it?

Shawn: Yes.

Keith: It's my favorite way to eat pizza. Well, now the whole pizza tastes that way. Here, try a slice.

Shawn: Hey, this pizza without cheese is good. Cool!

I merely let Shawn know that our way was a perfectly normal way to eat pizza. About one month later, Shawn, his mom, and I were planning another night out.

Shawn: Hey, Uncle Keith, can we order pizza again, the way you do? Mom won't order it that way.

Keith: Sure. Say, next time you and your mom order pizza, ask her to order half with cheese and half without. That way you both can have pizza the way you like it.

Shawn: Great idea. Did you hear that, Mom?

Mom (rolling her eyes): Yes, I heard that.

Getting children to try new foods requires a bit of finesse. But in a lot of cases you don't need to tell them about the substitution because they may not even notice.

Mental Preparation

Be Consistent

Whenever you place your hand over a fire, you get burned. Children learn these kinds of lessons fast. Fire is always consistent. You will never place your hand over a burning flame and discover that you did not get scorched. Teaching your child new eating habits also requires consistency. Although listening to your children whine their protests may be tough, do not let their complaints deter you! The bottom line is that all children require, want, and need consistency.

They may resist, cry, throw a temper tantrum, or do one of the many things that make a child a child; but you have worked hard to set rules and guidelines for lifetime weight control, and now you must be consistent. Let your kids know that your way is the way it is going to be and that the whole family will now adopt your new guidelines. But beware: Carefully consider the guidelines you have set down. It's important to lay down rules that are sensible ones to which your family can adhere. Don't set goals that will go by the wayside after two or three weeks. If you tell your kids that meals will be eaten at home and there will be no more fast food, be prepared to stick with that decision. If you tell your son, "No dessert tonight, Honey," don't change your mind ten minutes later. Withholding a sweet in this case is not the same thing as depriving him of food as a form of punishment. It is part of the rules you have established governing the frequency of desserts for your family. Don't permit your child to eat dinner in front of the TV one night and then declare it off limits the next. Personally, I don't believe that kids should ever be allowed to eat their meals in front of the television. Eating should be a singular activity.

Many children's weight problems stem from inconsistent eating patterns and verbal cues created by the parents. Mealtimes, as with other times—homework, television, nap times—need to be consistent. You can't tell your daughter that she needs to lose weight and then order pizza (with cheese) a few minutes later. And you can't complain about her lack of activity while confiding to your friend how much you hate to exercise. Remember, the ultimate payoff for your consistency in adhering to your own guidelines is a child who no longer has a weight problem.

Model Good Eating Habits

Your plans will not always go smoothly. Mistakes are going to happen with your weight control program just as they do in any other important area of life. But you can always pick up where you left off and go forward. Don't be surprised when frustration takes on a whole new level of meaning for you as you attempt to help your child lose weight. Like any other part of parenting, helping your child to eat properly is a twenty-four-hour job.

One of the best predictors for a child's success in weight loss is how effective as role models the parents are. Being a good role model involves taking the time yourself to be more physically active, eat healthily and prepare low fat foods. Eating habits are passed down by parents. If you go out to dinner and order pizza or a hamburger and fries, don't expect your son to order a grilled dry chicken breast! Although my mom used to say, "Do as I say and not as I do," I always did whatever she was doing. In other words, you cannot order a hot fudge sundae while explaining to your son why he can't.

Lay Down Your Plan

Part of the plan should be for the entire family to eat meals together on a regular basis. It's a good idea to delegate some of the responsibilities of food preparation, making sure to involve the kids. Let them set the table or do the dishes. If one parent has to work late, the other one can still sit down with the children at the designated meal time. Post your shopping list on the refrigerator and have everyone add to it. Whatever plan you decide on, involve the whole family and try to incorporate it as a part of your normal routine.

You may wonder why I reiterate the idea of sitting down as a family and eating together. There's more to it than just helping your child stay healthy. Researchers at the Cincinnati Children's Hospital Center studied 527 teenagers to find out whether there was a connection between certain family and lifestyle characteristics and mental health. They discovered that adolescents who ate dinner with their parents five times a week or more were less likely to be on drugs, depressed, or in trouble with the law. These same kids were more likely to do better in school.

The conclusion is that children do better in school and in society when they live in families that spend more time together, with parents who are more involved with their children. Children who are left alone or come home to an empty house tend to feel isolated. If you've read this far, you obviously care about your child's welfare. Thus, even if you're a single parent or both you and your spouse work, you can see that having a truly healthy child depends on your presence at the dinner table.

Time for a Family Meeting

Set up a family conference to discuss your family's new eating program. The conversation should be focused on the health of the family, not the weight of a particular child. I cannot emphasize strongly enough how important it is that neither you, nor any member of your family, zero in on the overweight child. By telling your daughter, for example, that she is the reason for the new eating program, you are making her responsible for its success. That is unfair, and it is sure to increase her stress, which will probably show up in sneaky snacking later.

Solicit Support from Extended Family Members

Call grandparents, the babysitter, and anyone else who has close contact with your overweight son. Meet with them and describe in confidence the challenges facing your family and the solutions you are implementing for your son's benefit. Ask them for their support, and emphasize the point made above about not singling out a particular family member as the reason for the new weight control program.

If you discover that some family members are not supporting the new eating plan, don't take the chance that your overweight son may be influenced by them. Provide him with healthy snacks as substitutes for fat-rich snacks he will encounter outside the home.

Even the best laid plans can go astray if your overweight son gives in to the influence of peer pressure to scuttle the new eating program. You may need to limit your son's contact with other children who are negative influences. This may involve painting a picture for him of what he will look like by adopting a new philosophy of eating. Children need solid goals they can visualize in order to pledge their determination.

Give Your Child Choices

Giving children food choices so they can feel a sense of control over their eating habits is another good strategy. Start by giving your daughter a choice between two healthy options each night. For example, you could offer a turkey burger with yam chips or a low fat Sloppy Joe. Giving her the decision of which meal to eat transfers responsibility to her for her dietary habits. Children learn quickly that they can take different actions by making choices. Realizing that they are the ones rowing the boat leads to a sense of personal power. It is a truism that when children learn to make healthier food choices, eventually their choices will fall on the positive side of the better/bad equation.

Find New Rewards

Food is fuel. It should never be used as a reward for good eating habits. But what is an appropriate reward? The best rewards are your compliments and your encouragement. Tell your daughter repeatedly how special she is, how proud you are of her accomplishments, and she will feel compelled to continue her behavior. You can never give a child too many compliments. In fact, the more sincere your compliments are, the more you will see her self-confidence and pride in herself grow.

Other rewards might include a video or computer game, model airplane, book, or collector's stamp. Maybe it's a trip to the zoo with some friends or a whole day at the movies. Whatever you decide on as a reward, please don't offer money to your kids; it sends the wrong message. If you offer money, a child will do whatever it takes to get the money even if it means skipping meals and going hungry. Her focus becomes the reward itself rather than changing for life her undesirable eating habits. Here's what you can expect if you offer money in return for weight loss: You'll be out fifty bucks and your daughter will gain back every pound she has lost and more. The difference between handing your child money and buying a special gift is that many children understand a love language that revolves around gifts. A gift shows your daughter that you appreciate her enough to take time to select something she will like, because she's special, not because she lost weight. Money doesn't have as much meaning as a well-wrapped present or a special occasion. Also, if cash is used as an incentive your daughter may begin using her weight as a bargaining point to get more money: "I'll lose five pounds for twenty dollars." If you fall for this gambit, I guarantee that her lost five pounds will return like a bird flying home, while your money flies away like a migrating bird.

Praise and Acceptance

Always praise your child. Let him know how proud you are; give him a hug or a pat on the back every chance you get. Encourage him, support him, and try your best to listen. Positive reinforcement will prompt your son to repeat the behaviors that you praise. A child who doesn't receive positive feedback may resort to weight gain just to get your attention.

I cannot overemphasize that a parent who is a positive role model and encourages a child will be amazed at the changes that occur. Think about when you were young. Was there someone in your life whom you could run to and tell about something really exciting that happened to you? Chances are that special person was your encourager. Encouragers are positive people who want us to be happy and successful. They boost our morale when we are down and light up a room when they walk in. Be this kind of role model for your child. It all begins with the way you reflect unconditional acceptance of your child. Test your own childhood memories to discover the character-building value of encouragement and respect you received from the person in your life you trusted with your accomplishments.

Give Your Child Lots of Attention

Kids crave attention and they will do just about anything to get it. If doing good things doesn't get Mom's attention, they may resort to doing bad things. Let's face it: Bad things often get more attention than good things. This is why it's so important for you to recognize when your child does good things.

Giving a child attention doesn't mean feeding her every time she asks for food. In fact, a lot of childhood weight gain stems from a parent's desire to avoid taking time out for her child. It's much easier to hand a crying child a cookie than find out what's really wrong. It's easier to have eight-year-old Suzy watch TV, than get in your way while you're doing the dishes. But it's a mistake to substitute food or folly for a child's time spent with you. A child who spends lots of time with a parent develops positive self-esteem. Take the time to listen to your child and play with her. And remember not to use food as a toy or a pacifier!

Be Careful about What You Say

Part of your plan must include a commitment never to make unfavorable comments about another person's physical appearance, especially his weight. A child who witnesses such casual judgments cannot help but apply your criticism to himself if he is overweight. Inevitably, though he may never mention it to you, his conclusion is, "Mom doesn't like fat people, and I'm fat."

Shift the Conversation to Your Child's Positive Attributes

Pay attention when your daughter expresses discomfort about her appearance. Sit down with her, listen, and be as supportive as possible. Don't dismiss her feelings by saying, "You're just imagining things." If she says, "My stomach is too big," or "I'm fat," don't agree with her. She doesn't want confirmation, she wants comfort and verbal cuddling. Try shifting the conversation to her positive attributes, areas in which she excels. It's important for you to help her identify her personal strengths and establish a strong personal focus rather than accepting as gospel the negative remarks of her peers.

Take Your Child for a Walk

It amazes me how many times I see adults walking their dogs, but I never see them walking with their children. Kids love and need physical activity. Choose something your child enjoys, whether it's karate, roller skating, jumping rope, biking, basketball, or skipping. Kids want to be moving. Associate exercise with positive feelings, and don't use exercise as a form of punishment.

It may help if you make exercise a family affair. Some fitness facilities have planned activities for kids. While your kids are doing their thing, you can get in your own good workout. Exercise goals should be set, and when met by your children, make sure they are rewarded—but never with food! Most of the children I have worked with seem to do better with a variety of exercises as opposed to only one form. By varying the activities, you prevent boredom. Above all, a child needs to know that exercise can be—and is—fun!

Give Your Child Creative Activities

Get your kids engaged in activities that relieve boredom. There are so many ways: Rollerblading, team sports, puzzles, arts and crafts, reading, listening to music, or taking a walk. And be sure to give them as many positive strokes as possible to reinforce their participation in the activity; they build a child's self-esteem. Positive strokes reinforce productive behaviors and increase a child's set of positive attributes. Then, he is able to call on his pool of resources to override any negative influences.

Reduce Your Child's Television Watching

I can't stress this enough. Many kids snack on high fat junk food while watching television or playing video games. On average, children watch between twenty-two and twenty-five hours of television each week. If a child sits in front of the TV for twenty-five hours a week, she is exposed to an onslaught of commercials aimed directly at her. Television advertising promotes kids' food consumption, which should not be surprising given that more than 11,000 high-calorie junk food commercials a year are aimed at children. Here's a sobering statistic: Obesity increases 2 percent for every hour per week a child sits in front of a television set.

The role that television plays in childhood obesity has been extensively documented. Not only does television take kids away from other activities that burn calories, the commercials bombard them with mixed messages concerning food. The American Academy of Pediatrics suggests that parents limit their child's television viewing to a maximum of one or two hours a day. Reducing your child's television watching is one of the most important areas over which you have control.

Do not ever give in to the erroneous assumption that watching TV together is a bonding experience for families. Turn off the TV and play a game. Getting involved and spending time with your child will reduce those of his eating habits that stem from lone-liness or feelings of not being cared for. That's right! Whether they realize it or not, many children use TV as a substitute for the attention of their parents. Your presence and involvement with your kids will replace their urge to eat. A helpful hint: Spend as much time with your child as he will allow, because when he gets older you will be begging him to spend time with you!

Spending more time with your kids, in conjunction with less television watching, encourages discussion and gives your child a chance to be heard. No kid grows up resenting his parents for limiting his television watching time. In fact, he may thank you for it one day!

I think it is worth repeating here: Obesity increases by 2 percent for every hour per week a child sits in front of a television set!

The Goal Is Progress, Not Perfection

One cold hard fact about real-world eating is that there will be occasional flat tires. There will be holidays, birthdays, family parties, and friends hanging out—times when a child may slide. But this is okay. I want you to understand that the goal of the program presented here is progress, not perfection.

Ironically, bad choices must be part of your child's program. If you place your daughter on a diet and expect her to follow it to the letter, you have begun laying down a series of barriers that she will face for a lifetime. For your child to succeed, bad choices must be managed rather than omitted. Cutting out all of her favorite foods will only lead to stronger and stronger cravings that can develop a life all their own. While most nutri-tionists avoid using the word "relapse," they recognize that in a dieting regimen of depri-vation, your daughter may revert to previous bad habits. Be prepared. Having a plan is a lot like conducting a fire drill. We have fire drills not because there is an actual fire, but in order that should one occur we will know what to do. Understanding the root cause of bingeing is one way to help your daughter overcome the hopelessness and helplessness she may feel whenever one does occur.

The expectation of perfection is an unbearable pressure on a child. Your son may develop the sense that he can never live up to your expectations. This will cause you to lose patience when your expectations are not being met. Try lowering your expectations and realize that kids require constant reminders before they fully comprehend something new. I have never met a child who did what a parent asked the first time. It takes patience, understanding, and time, on both your part and your child's, to understand that the old rules have changed.

Teaching Good Habits

Successfully helping your child lose body fat requires more than knowledge about food and exercise. It also requires good habits. Unfortunately, most people overlook the importance of good habits concerning food and exercise. But positive habits can be taught or learned at any age. With the proper habits, eating and exercise goals are a lot easier to attain and manage.

For the past sixteen years, I have carried a cooler of food to work with me. I forgot it one day but didn't realize my oversight until I arrived at the office. At that point, I knew it would be a rough day. I take two breaks each afternoon, from 12:30 to 1:00, and from 3:30 to 4:00. During these breaks, I normally return phone calls and eat. This time, because I hadn't brought any food, when 12:30 arrived, I ran downstairs to the deli on the first floor. This particular deli doesn't serve low fat food, so I made a Better Bad Choice: a hamburger with no mayonnaise or cheese. By the time I finished eating, it was already 1:00. I ran upstairs to my office to return phone calls but my next client had already arrived. My stress level went up a notch because I didn't have a chance to return the calls.

Rationalizing and Justifying

The food I ate at lunch didn't satisfy me for long. By the time 3:30 rolled around, I was starving. Once again, I ran down to the deli, but this time I began to justify and rationalize eating other things. I grabbed a bag of pretzels and a banana along with my burger. As I stood there in line, I eyed a display of chocolate chip cookies. Although tempted, I resisted this "trigger." By the time I got back upstairs it was 4:00. As soon as I walked in the door, my next appointment was waiting, so once again, I could not return any calls. Add two more notches on the stress scale. At 6:00 that evening, I was still at work and now had one and a half hours of calls to return. I finally left the office about 7:30.

Feeling stressed out, hungry and tired, I began to justify and rationalize once again. I convinced myself that I could skip my workout and make it up later in the week. On the way home, I stopped for a chicken breast and baked potato. I was almost out of the restaurant when two chocolate chip cookies beckoned me over to the dessert counter. Although I had resisted the chocolate chip cookies earlier in the day, I couldn't refuse them again.

My usual evening routine once I get home includes writing for two hours in order to keep up with all my commitments: a radio and television show, monthly newsletter, and articles for various monthly magazines. Under normal circumstances, I enjoy these two hours. However, I dreaded the time on this particular evening.

Let's look at the series of dominoes that fell because one habit—taking my lunch cooler—was interrupted:

1. My eating plan was off for the day and I ate foods I normally wouldn't eat.
2. My energy suffered.
3. Cravings for other foods surfaced.
4. I missed my workout.
5. My stress level increased throughout the day.
6. I didn't have any free time.

Here's the point of my story: By spending a mere twenty minutes each morning putting together my cooler, I feel in control of my day and in control of food. It helps to keep me on my self-imposed time schedule, gives me lots of energy, allows me to leave work at a decent hour and exercise at my allotted time, reduces cravings for unhealthy foods, and it really pleases my wife when I arrive home in a good mood!

If you can help your child to establish and maintain a disciplined routine when it comes to food, you will give him an important tool for long-term weight control success.

For those of you who say, "I can't afford an extra twenty minutes to spend in the morning fixing my child's lunch," my response is, "You can't afford not to."

Don't Let Your Child Buy Lunch at School

The way I remember it, when I was young most kids brought their lunch to school. But at some point, our parents made the decision to quit packing our lunches and gave us lunch money instead—a really big mistake. Suppose your daughter has always taken a fairly healthy, low fat lunch to school: a tuna sandwich, baked potato chips, and an apple. If all of a sudden you stop sending her lunch with her, at first she might try to order a similar one in the school cafeteria. Unfortunately, most schools serve incredibly high fat lunches, which makes eating healthy not very practical. More than likely, before long your daughter will be eating pizza, burgers, and ice cream. By teaching your child to carry her own healthy lunch, you will establish a habit that will be easier for her to maintain as an adult.

Schedule Your Child's Playtime

Another habit I learned long ago is to bring my workout clothes with me to work; otherwise, I will never make it to the gym. After fighting rush hour traffic for forty minutes, the last thing I want to do when I finally get home is get back on the road. Maybe you prefer to exercise before work. Whatever works for you is okay as long as you do it consistently. Just as you schedule your child's study time, be sure to schedule play time or exercise time as well. Be consistent with your son's physical activity and it will become a routine part of his day. Enrolling a child in sports, for example, is a great way to structure his play time. Once he becomes accustomed to the routine of regular practices and games, your son will look forward to this organized activity and it will become a regular part of his life. In addition, he will be associating with other kids who are athletic. These associations in turn will allow him to maintain friendships with other healthy kids.

Habits Are Learned

Most children have a routine they perform every day. A routine is a series of habitual behaviors. When your daughter gets ready for school, she probably proceeds in almost the exact same order each day. She probably walks the same way to school every morning, and may even leave the house at exactly the same time. Good habits, whether in getting ready for school or planning meals, are a vital part of any successful eating program. For example, I shop at least once a week, every week, and then cook enough food to last two or three days. These simple habits allow me to have all the necessary foods available to cook adequate meals. Helping children lose weight depends on your ability to teach them habits that will lead them toward their goal, not take them away from it.

Ten Good Habits to Help Your Child
Lose Weight the Right Way

1. Keep an ongoing shopping list and shop at least once a week.
2. Develop as many great tasting recipes as possible. (The recipes in the back of this book are a good place to start.)
3. Set up play time and help your child become more active.
4. Prepare large quantities of food ahead of time.
5. Pack your child's food in a lunch kit or cooler. Let her pick one that will be fun to carry to school.
6. Teach your child to say no to activities that he really doesn't have time to do.
7. Try to identify your child's high-risk eating places and avoid them. But if fast food was the norm, allow her to have it occasionally.
8. Pack a snack in your child's cooler for the midafternoon.
9. Try to set up regular mealtimes and stick to them. This helps a child avoid hunger and cravings for junk food.
10. Limit eating out in restaurants to two times a week, if possible.

Determining an Ideal Caloric Intake

No matter how many times I recommend that you should not be a calorie counter, you may still wonder how the eating program I am suggesting translates into the calories your child should be consuming on a daily basis. The good news is that you do not need to count calories every day. But you should understand the caloric *range* within which you should strive to stay for your child. Here's a good rule of thumb: A child's daily caloric intake should equal her ideal weight times fifteen. So if your daughter's ideal weight is eighty pounds, she should be eating about 1200 calories per day (80 x 15 = 1200). Calculate her caloric intake before starting this program to get an idea of how many calories a day she is currently eating. A calorie counting book can be purchased from any local bookstore. To begin, try to keep an accurate record of everything your child eats over the course of one week. Add up the total calories for the day each evening. At the end of seven days, add all the daily totals together and divide by seven. This will let you know the average number of calories your daughter is eating each day.

Perhaps she has been diagnosed as being overweight. After charting the calories, you find that she has been consuming an average of 2,100 calories a day and weighs 110 pounds. In this case, it's apparent that 2,100 calories a day is too much for her. Begin to implement Better Bad Choices, which in turn will decrease her fat and calorie intake. After she has been on the eating program a couple of weeks, recheck her caloric intake as you did before. You should be able to see a healthy decrease in overall calories and fat.

A child's appetite, not you, should dictate how much of the better foods she is eating. By coupling Better Bad Choices with an increased activity level, your daughter will now grow into her weight.

Weight Maintenance

Many parents have told me that having their kids lose weight was the easy part; the really hard part was helping them maintain the loss. Again, let me stress that the goal of this program is to establish lifelong habits of healthy eating and exercise. The only way that weight loss or any normal weight will be maintained is by developing the mindset that the eating philosophy proposed here is forever. The good news is that your child will not only have the tools to make healthy choices, but he will be enjoying the food choices so much that he will never want to abandon them.

Remember, weight control is not a quick fix. Attaining the goal of eating healthy is a continuous process, one that involves being open to trying new foods and making Better Bad Choices. Progress, not perfection, is our goal. Healthy eating is actually quite simple.

What Do I Do First?

Begin by planning the family shopping list. I have included a suggested shopping list to make things easy and help you get started. Of course, you should feel free to add or delete items according to your family's needs. This list is designed for a family of three. So if your family is bigger, you may need to double or even triple some of the items. Certain items may not need to be purchased every week. And some of the spices may last several months before restocking. Feeding your family natural, wholesome foods will become easier with shopping practice!

A quick review of the basics: Center your child's diet around chicken or turkey breast, fresh fish, baked potatoes, rice, whole grains, vegetables, and fresh fruit. Processed, refined foods often contain hidden fats, sugars, and sodium. Avoid luncheon meats, canned foods, and packaged foods as much as possible. We all have a tendency in today's fast-paced world to reach for whatever is fastest and easiest, which, unfortunately, often leads to eating lower quality foods. Fast food, eating in restaurants, and buying frozen, packaged meals can rapidly destroy your child's health.

Shopping Savvy

One of the most important aspects of eating healthy is shopping for healthy foods on a regular basis. Successful people understand that shopping at least once a week allows them to stock their cupboards with healthy low fat foods. When hunger strikes, they have healthy choices available to satisfy their appetite. People who don't shop regularly are putting themselves in a high risk situation. In other words, once their cupboards run bare, they'll be out the door hunting for their next meal.

A basic rule of thumb for shopping healthy is to purchase most of your foods from the outer perimeter of the supermarket. The inner aisles are mainly stocked with processed foods. The outer sections display the natural, unprocessed foods. For example, fruits, vegetables, meats, seafood and dairy products usually line the outer four walls of the supermarket, because they require refrigeration. The central aisles typically contain non-perishable foods like canned goods, cookies, crackers, soups, etc. So make it a point to spend most of your shopping in the areas where the natural foods are found. Shopping for natural, fresh foods is a vital part of preparing low fat meals.

Another thing to remember while shopping is that variety is important. If you eat the same foods all the time, or worse yet, if you don't develop good tasting recipes that you enjoy, you will end up developing strong cravings and bingeing. Begin by rotating in one new low fat recipe per week. After several weeks, you and your family will be shocked at how easy the transition from high fat to low fat eating is.

The following shopping list is fairly complete, and everything on the list is under 20 percent fat. This list isn't supposed to be used as a strict guideline, but rather is designed to help you develop your own weekly shopping list. The list includes groups of food that will help you maximize the variety in your daily diet. To get the most out of your shopping list, photocopy it, and place a copy on your refrigerator. When you get low or use up the last of a particular food, just circle that item on the list. When it's time to shop, your list will instantly show you exactly what you need to buy for the upcoming week.

The One-Week Shopping List
(Select quantities that meet the needs of your family)
Beverages
diet soda
Crystal Light or NutraSweet Kool Aid
decaffeinated tea bags to make iced tea
Quest
sparkling waters

Snacks
NutraSweet Jell-O
NutraSweet pudding
frozen yogurt or fat-free ice cream
baked potato chips or tortilla chips
Guiltless Gourmet popcorn
rice cakes
pretzels*

Breads
whole wheat English muffins*
lite whole wheat bread*
pita bread*
    (Note: English muffins, pita, and bread can be frozen to prolong shelf life.)
crackers*
tortillas*
quick cooking oatmeal or grits
low sugar cereal (try unfrosted Shredded Wheat, Cheerios, etc.)
pasta (spaghetti, linguine, fettuccine)*

Condiments
dill relish
low sugar jam
fat-free mayonnaise
low sodium soy sauce

---

*Although these foods are healthy and low in fat, they should be limited because they are made from refined flour.

low sodium teriyaki sauce
mustard
catsup
Tabasco Jalapeño Sauce (the green Tabasco is spicy but not too hot)
Healthy Choice BBQ sauce
Knorr vegetable soup mix
fat-free salad dressings like Ranch, Thousand Island, and Italian
picante sauce
cooking spray

Canned Goods
soup
chicken broth
whole tomatoes
Hunt's tomato sauces
tomato paste (Try Hunt's Mexican, garlic, or Italian flavored tomato pastes)

Dairy
skim milk
fat-free yogurt
fat-free cheese (cheddar, mozzarella or Swiss. They make these grated and in slices—
buy both)
fat-free Parmesan cheese
fat-free cream cheese
fat-free sour cream
fat-free Promise
eggs or Egg Beaters (frozen)

Fruits
pineapple in its own juice
unsweetened applesauce
fresh fruits your child likes

Grains and Beans
popcorn for air popper
rice (try different varieties like brown rice, basmati, jasmine, Texmati, wild rice)
canned black beans
canned kidney beans (choose the reduced salt variety)
canned black-eyed peas

lentils
barley
bulgur, millet, or couscous (quick and simple to prepare, and tasty!)
flour

Lean Meats
skinless chicken breast
skinless turkey breast
ground turkey breast
shrimp (from the meat counter)
imitation crab
scallops
water packed tuna
(Note: All meats can be frozen and thawed just before cooking.)

Herbs and Spices
(Check your current supply of these and purchase only the ones you may need.)
baking powder
basil
Cajun seasoning
celery salt
cinnamon
cocoa powder
cornstarch
cumin
dill
minced garlic (ready to use from the jar)
garlic salt
minced onion
oregano
parsley
pepper
rosemary
salt
thyme

Vegetables (avoid canned; frozen is okay and avoids waste)
celery
lettuce

tomatoes
onions
bell peppers
baking potatoes or yams
carrots, corn, peas (or other fresh or frozen vegetables that your child likes)
water chestnuts
shredded potatoes or hash browns (choose the 100 percent potato variety with no added fat)

Meal Balance

A growing child requires additional nutrients. The best way to ensure that your child gets what she needs is by serving balanced meals the majority of the time. A good rule of thumb is to imagine her plate divided in thirds. Place a vegetable on one third, a small portion of protein on the other third, and a large serving of complex carbohydrate on the other third. Naturally, not all meals will be laid out like this. Example: If you are serving lasagna for dinner, the plate should have a nice serving of lasagna, along with a dinner salad and fat-free dressing. If you are serving Hawaiian chicken for dinner, also place a serving of rice on the plate, with the chicken breast on top, and pineapple pico de gallo on top of this. Although the meal may not be served in thirds each time, the concept is to have a serving of each food on the plate.

An unbalanced meal would be one in which the plate is filled with nothing but carbohydrates. Example: A plate covered with vegetables and rice but no protein would not be a balanced meal. Not every single meal has to be balanced. Just keep in mind that the majority of them should be.

Sample Eating Program

Now Show Me

Let's look at a sample menu plan to give you an idea of the best way to lay out your child's eating program. This sample menu is not etched in stone. It's merely a guideline to help you with meal layout and introduce nutritious nibbling. Be creative and use the recipes to add variety to your child's daily eating program.

Breakfast: low sugar cereal with skim milk
Midmorning: fresh fruit
Lunch: chicken salad sandwich on lite whole wheat bread and a piece of fresh fruit
Midafternoon: yogurt, oats and raisins
Dinner: turkey burger with yam chips, glass of skim milk

Notice that I included a mini-meal in the middle of the afternoon. When you mix the yogurt with uncooked oatmeal and raisins, the oats absorb the moisture from the yogurt, and the raisins become more plump. This little snack is sweet and full of nutrients, and provides a lot of energy during the middle of the day. Other snacks might be a fat-free cheese sandwich on lite bread or a small root beer float made with lite frozen yogurt and diet root beer. Make it one of your goals to discover as many great-tasting, low fat recipes as possible that your child enjoys.

Chapter 6

Fats, Carbohydrates and Proteins

The Food Pyramid

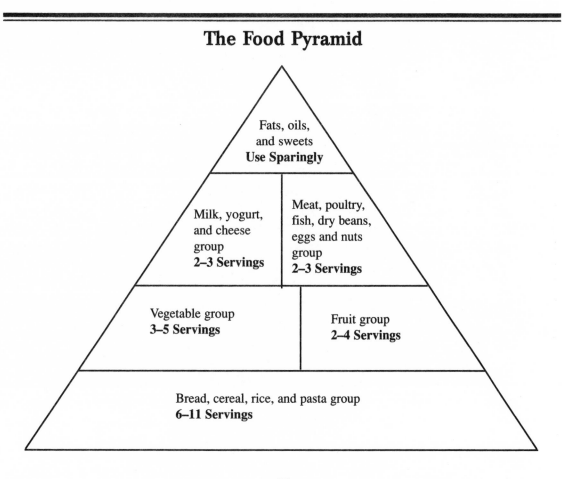

Fats, oils,
and sweets
Use Sparingly

Milk, yogurt,
and cheese
group
2–3 Servings

Meat, poultry,
fish, dry beans,
eggs and nuts
group
2–3 Servings

Vegetable group
3–5 Servings

Fruit group
2–4 Servings

Bread, cereal, rice, and pasta group
6–11 Servings

In 1957, in an effort to establish guidelines to help the average American eat a nutritionally balanced diet, the United States Department of Agriculture (USDA) created the concept of basic food groups. They devised four categories—fruits and vegetables, breads and cereals, meat, and dairy— and recommended daily serving amounts for each. After many years, the USDA declared the four basic food groups obsolete and replaced the previous guidelines with a new food guide pyramid. Ironically, the food guide pyramid with which our children in the 1990s are familiar is almost identical to the food group guidelines that we adults learned in the 1950s.

The pyramid shape is well-suited for the USDA's new guidelines, because it represents visually the idea of building a healthy diet on a solid foundation of highly nutritious foods, and eating less of foods that aren't good for you.

At the base of the food pyramid are the foods that the USDA suggests we eat abundantly, such as bread, pasta, cereal and rice. They recommend six to eleven servings per day from this group. On top of this foundation, The USDA recommends that we consume three to five servings per day from the vegetable group and two or three servings of fruit. Wow! Already this seems like a lot of food!

Two more food groups sit directly above the fruits and vegetables. One is the dairy group, including milk, yogurt and cheese, and the other group is for meat, poultry, fish, dry beans, eggs and nuts. The USDA recommends that we eat two or three servings per day from each of these groups. At the top of the pyramid sit the foods that we should eat the least—fats, oils, and sweets.

Does the New Pyramid Represent a Good Diet for Your Child?

Although the new pyramid builds on the proper foundation of grains, rice, vegetables, and fruits, all of which are healthy, a crucial flaw in the USDA's recommendations could sabotage your entire healthy eating plan. The USDA made a big mistake when it failed to group red meats and high fat dairy products—both of which contain saturated fat, the worst kind—with the other fats at the top of the pyramid. If nothing else, they should be included in the "use sparingly" group. When whole milk and cheese, both high fat foods, are grouped with low fat milk products, it implies that all milk products are equally healthy, which is simply not true. Similarly, to list red meat right alongside poultry, fish, and beans may lead people to believe that red meat is as healthy as chicken or fish. Wrong!

If we followed the USDA's advice and fed our families two or three servings of red meat each day (about nine ounces), we would consume a lot of saturated fat and cholesterol. As I have already mentioned, you should omit as much red meat and high fat dairy products from your child's diet as possible.

Part of the reason that high fat dairy foods and red meat are grouped with poultry, fish, and beans is because when the meat group was first introduced during the 1950s, all proteins were thought to be alike. Back then, we were unaware of many of the adverse effects of fat on our health. Today, however, no self-respecting nutritionist would claim that red meat is as healthy as beans. The nutritional values of these two foods are very different and should not be treated equally. It would make far more sense to group beans with grains, pasta and rice, and to list red meat along with fats, oils, and sweets.

Politics and Food Don't Digest Well Together

Another important reason for the odd grouping of high fat foods involves politics. The main purpose of the USDA is to protect and promote the U.S. livestock industry. If the USDA announced that Americans should eat red meat and dairy products "sparingly," it would be defeating its own purpose of creating markets for U.S. livestock products. The USDA has a conflict of interest: The agency subsidizes special-interest agricultural groups, while at the same time suggesting how we, as a nation, should eat. It's a fair question to ask whether the food pyramid represents what the meat and dairy producers would like for Americans to eat, or what is actually best for our health. What would the USDA recommend if it were not also supporting the meat and dairy industry?

Because the food pyramid is not based on consistently sound nutritional principles, my program doesn't follow the USDA's guidelines. If you follow the plan that I am proposing, your children will lose weight and become healthier by limiting fats, particularly red meats and high fat dairy products.

Fat Facts

Remember the days when no one paid attention to fat? And who ever worried about the types of fat we were eating? We smeared butter on our toast, used it heavily in our recipes, and fried our chicken and doughnuts in lard. Today almost all recipes can be modified to include little or no fat, but there is so much misleading advice that it seems as if the average person should have a degree in nutrition before he or she embarks on preparing a meal. Saturated fat, polyunsaturated fat, monounsaturated fat—what's a cook to do? Cooking without fat is actually quite simple if you understand a few basics.

What Are Fats?

There are three main types of fat: saturated, polyunsaturated, and monounsaturated. These come in solid forms such as butter, cheese, and shortening, or in a liquid form such as oil. All fats contain nine calories per gram, compared to four calories per gram for proteins or carbohydrates.

Saturated fat is found mainly in foods that come from animals, such as meat, eggs, butter, and cheese. The only two saturated fats that don't come from an animal are coconut oil and palm oil. Saturated fat impacts a child's level of cholesterol, and saturated fat has been linked to a higher incidence of coronary heart disease, cancer, and obesity—a good reason to limit it.

Beef and pork are the primary sources of saturated fat in the average American's diet, supplying 38 percent of our daily saturated fat and about 35 percent of our daily cholesterol. Your child should be eating less than two hundred milligrams of cholesterol per day. Research has shown that people who consume high amounts of animal fat have higher rates of colon and prostate cancer. One study found that people who ate red meat once a day were twice as likely to develop colon cancer. You don't need to eliminate red meat from your family's diet, but it does make sense to limit how often you serve it.

Saturated fats cause your child's body to produce excessive amounts of cholesterol. Coconut oil and palm oil don't contain any cholesterol themselves, but they stimulate the body to produce high levels of cholesterol. Chips and snack foods that are fried in these oils should be limited.

Unsaturated fats are different from saturated fats because they don't cause an elevation of cholesterol and don't play a role in heart disease. Unsaturated fats are most often found in plants and seafood. Examples of monounsaturated fats include canola oil and olive oil. Examples of polyunsaturated fats include sunflower oil and corn oil.

Don't Be Confused about Fat

The only way to determine whether or not a food is low in fat is to calculate the percentage of the total calories that come from fat. Don't be fooled by the number of grams of fat listed on a product's label. In an effort to give us what they think we want, manufacturers have developed marketing techniques that can make high fat foods appear to have low numbers of fat grams.

Unfortunately, the Food and Drug Administration (FDA) has chosen not to include the percentage of fat on labels for the simple reason that many consumers would avoid products if they knew the percentage of total calories that come from fat. Although it may appear to be a hassle to do arithmetic every time you shop, if you're serious about improving your child's diet, carry a small calculator with you to the store.

The Fat Formula

To determine the percentage of fat within a food, locate the "calories from fat" listed on the label. Divide this number by the total calories per serving. You may be shocked to discover that many seemingly low fat foods actually derive more than half of their total calories from fat. Let's use the fat formula on the label from a package of popular luncheon meat.

Amount Per Serving

Calories 14   Calories from Fat 4

The label we have chosen is a brand of "lean ham" listing calories from fat as 4. In this example, total calories per serving are 14. Now let's plug this into our formula: Calories from fat (4) divided by total calories (14) equals percentage of calories from fat.

4/14 = percent of fat (29%)

Using the fat formula, we know that the luncheon meat derives 29 percent of its calories from fat, which is a high percentage of fat for a food.

Let's try another label. If a product's label lists the calories from fat as 150 and the total calories are 420, what is the percentage of calories from fat?

150 calories from fat/420 calories = 36 percent from fat

As you can see, the above example gets 36 percent of its caloric content from fat. This is certainly a high fat food.

Try to Keep Most of the Food You Choose under 20 Percent Fat

The golden rule of healthy eating for the whole family is to build your menu around foods that are under 20 percent fat. *If each individual food your daughter eats is under 20 percent fat, her overall diet will also be under 20 percent fat.* This doesn't mean that she can never eat a food that contains 50 percent fat, but higher fat foods should be served only occasionally. All red meat is higher than 20 percent fat. Consequently, red meat should be rotated into your child's diet occasionally, maybe once a week or so. To help you with your meal planning, I've included a list of better, leaner cuts of beef in the appendix.

Why Is 20 Percent Fat the Magic Number?

For years, our government advised us that 30 percent or less of our calories should be from fat. But did you know that the 30 percent figure was chosen arbitrarily? The government knew that Americans were consuming an average of 40 percent of their calories in the form of fat. By setting the standard at 30 percent, the authorities hoped that more people would adhere to the lower guideline. Even though the experts knew that the optimum number for fat consumption was less than 20 percent of total calories, they picked a higher number that more people would presumably be able to reach. Go figure!

Does a Child Need Fats to Grow Up Healthy?

Believe it or not, almost every food contains some fat. Bananas contain fat; chicken or turkey breast contains fat; even vegetables contain fat. Fats are absolutely essential to a child's growth and development, but most kids' weight problems are caused by eating too much fat, too much sugar and too many calories. Let's be realistic. It's unlikely that your children will give up higher fat snacks and occasional high fat meals completely. A zero-fat diet is not the goal. The goal is to reduce your child's consumption of fat to 20 percent of total calories, which will provide enough fat to grow up healthy, but not enough to risk their health or cause a weight gain. Although most adults would benefit by eating 10 percent to 15 percent fat, for a growing child, eating too far below 20 percent fat may not be healthy.

Never, under any circumstances, cut fat out of the diet of an infant or toddler. During the early stages of development, fats aid in the building of almost every cell. Restricting the fat intake of a child under the age of two could cause health problems, because a low fat diet could possibly prevent growth and normal development, especially of the brain and nervous system. Children above the age of two, however, develop very healthy bodies on 20 percent or less fat. You don't have to cook differently for kids under two years old; *simply add a glass of whole milk* to their meal and they'll have all the fat they need.

What about Foods That Don't Have Labels?

In the appendix, I've included an easy reference guide of fat percentages for poultry, beef, pork, lamb, veal, and seafood, to help you with your shopping. I have also listed all the low fat meats that are good for your family in the Protein section of this chapter.

Are Certain Types of Fat Better Than Others?

Unlike saturated fats, unsaturated fats don't contribute to heart disease and elevated cholesterol. However, they do contribute to obesity, so you should limit these so-called healthy fats in your child's diet. Unsaturated fat comes in two types: monounsaturated and polyunsaturated. Polyunsaturated fats (safflower, corn, cottonseed, sunflower, and soybean oils) lower cholesterol levels slightly more than monounsaturated fats (olive and canola oils), but there are several characteristics of polyunsaturated fat that make it less desirable.

Polyunsaturated fats are more susceptible to oxidation, and oxidized fats appear to be responsible for clogging arteries. Feeding your child a lot of polyunsaturated fat could lay the building blocks for circulatory problems later in life. It often takes years for the effects of a poor diet to surface; cardiovascular disease doesn't happen overnight.

Although polyunsaturated fats reduce cholesterol levels in the bloodstream, they also reduce the amount of good cholesterol (HDL or high density lipid). Eating too many polyunsaturated fats can increase a child's risk of developing cancer. Studies have shown that lifetime consumption of monounsaturated fats is not harmful to humans. Populations in the Mediterranean have eaten large quantities of olive oil (monounsaturated fat) for decades and have suffered no negative consequences from this type of fat. Because there are no populations that have eaten high levels of polyunsaturated fat for long periods of time, it is not known what effects will result from a lifetime consumption of polyunsaturated fats.

Oil is a common source of fat. If you must cook with oil, try monounsaturated oils such as olive, high oleic safflower, high oleic sunflower, sesame, or canola. Studies have shown that monounsaturated oils can lower the bad cholesterol (LDL, or low density lipid) in your child's blood. These oils may actually reduce your child's risk of developing heart disease later in life.

Trans-Fatty Acids

To make oils solid and more stable so they can be used in baked goods and have a longer shelf life, food manufacturers hydrogenate oils by adding hydrogen atoms to soybean, corn, safflower, and other liquid oils. Unfortunately, hydrogenation can transform many of an oil's unsaturated fatty acids into trans-fatty acids, making the oil react more like a saturated fat. When trans-fatty acids are ingested, they react with the liver and raise blood serum cholesterol levels in almost exactly the same way as saturated fats. Although trans-fatty acids raise cholesterol levels to a lesser extent than saturated fats, they still are harmful—especially because their cholesterol-raising ability is hidden on the new food labels.

If you look on the side panel of almost any margarine box, you will see the words "partially hydrogenated oil" in the ingredient list. Partially hydrogenated oils contain trans-fatty acids. Margarine is a good example of a product that doesn't appear to contain any cholesterol, yet because it contains hidden trans-fatty acids, it causes an elevation of cholesterol in the bloodstream. No wonder you may be confused while shopping. Who would ever think that vegetable margarine would actually increase cholesterol levels? Although specific amounts of trans-fatty acids vary with each brand, tub margarines tend to have fewer than stick margarine. Kids who eat margarine instead of butter to prevent high cholesterol are not necessarily better off. A child above the age of three should limit all fat intake, including regular butter and margarine—so switch to light margarine.

Enough Fat Talk!

Don't be overwhelmed trying to keep all this fat information straight. If you can accomplish two easy-to-remember objectives, you won't need to worry about which fat is which:
- Reduce your child's total daily fat intake to below 20 percent of total calories.
- Restrict cholesterol consumption to less than two hundred milligrams per day.

If you select foods that contain less than 20 percent fat and limit the amount of red meat and fried foods that you serve, your child will automatically be eating a low-saturated-fat diet. Doesn't this seem simple enough?

Carbohydrates

Carbohydrates come in three varieties: monosaccharides, disaccharides, and poly-saccharides. Monosaccharide and disaccharide are fancy, twenty-five-cent words for simple sugars. Polysaccharides are complex carbohydrates, more commonly referred to as starches. Monosaccharides include glucose, fructose (fruit sugar), and galactose. Disaccharides include brown sugar, sucrose, corn syrup, maple syrup, honey, and lactose. Lactose, or milk sugar, is found in all dairy products such as milk, cheese, cottage cheese, and yogurt.

By refining a complex carbohydrate (like corn or rice), we can create sugars that are very similar to sucrose but sound much healthier. Don't be fooled. Even though corn syrup or rice syrup may sound healthy and complex, once the corn or rice is processed and refined, it loses its nutritional value. Corn syrup is nothing more than a simple sugar.

Simple sugars come in a variety of disguises and can be found in everything from pre-workout drinks, beverages, and baked goods, to frozen yogurt. For example, when you read the label on many health or energy bars, you will notice several forms of sugar. Many are loaded with sugars such as corn syrup, fructose, glucose, rice syrup, honey, brown sugar, or malt syrup. Manufacturers like to use these types of sugars because they sound as though they come from healthy foods. Don't make the mistake of thinking that these sugars are as healthy as the foods from which they are derived. (There'll be more on sugars later.)

The Function of Carbohydrates–Energy

The primary function of carbohydrates, both starches and sugars, is as an energy source for your child's body. All carbohydrates are broken down by the body into simple sugars, but many foods (such as potatoes, corn, rice, grains, and beans) consist of complex carbohydrates that are generally high in fiber, cholesterol free, low in fat (especially saturated fat), and full of vitamins and minerals. Carbohydrates contain four calories per gram, the same caloric value as protein, but unlike some high-protein foods such as meats and dairy products, complex carbohydrates are relatively low in fat.

Studies have shown that in countries where the diet is rich in complex carbohydrates, the risks of cancer, heart disease, and obesity are lower.

Keep your child away from a low-carbohydrate diet! If your son's diet is lacking in carbohydrates, his body will convert amino acids from within his muscles into energy, resulting in a loss of muscle, fatigue, weakness, and low energy. When your son's diet contains sufficient quantities of complex carbohydrates, his body will obtain most of its energy or fuel from the carbohydrates, rather than from protein. As a result, carbohydrates help prevent protein (amino acids) from being used as a source of fuel.

Complex Carbohydrates

Carbohydrates are perhaps the most misunderstood foods, because some children tolerate them very well—they can eat a lot and yet remain lean—while others seem to have a carbohydrate intolerance: Though they eat the same amount as other kids, they end up being overweight. This phenomenon can be explained by variations in human body chemistry.

Some complex carbohydrates are very low in fat and extremely healthy. Fresh or frozen vegetables, for example, are great for kids to eat. Do not serve canned vegetables, because the canning process results in excess sodium and a loss of nutrients. In general, complex carbohydrates that are very low in fat and wonderfully healthy tend to be unprocessed foods.

A child's body can store carbohydrates as fat, but one would have to eat a lot of these foods before they would be converted into body fat.

Healthy Low Fat Complex Carbohydrates

Barley	Corn tortillas	Peas
Beans	Cream of Wheat	Potatoes (all varieties)
Black-eyed peas	Kashi	Rice (all varieties)
Bread (lite)	Lentils	Rice cakes
Corn	Oatmeal	Yams

Certain Complex Carbohydrates May Slow Down Weight Loss

Not all complex carbohydrates will help your child lose weight. There is a big difference between eating healthy foods and eating healthy foods that will help your child become leaner. Although breads, pasta, crackers, and pretzels are all part of the carbohydrate family, they may slow down or stop your child's weight loss. Flour-based products are often healthy and low in fat, but the refining process alters the complex carbohydrates found in the wheat so that they more closely resemble simple sugars.

Consider this: There are four hundred calories in one cup of flour. Two cups of whole wheat grain were milled to make that one cup of flour. Because it took two cups of grain to make one cup of flour, the end product is twice as calorie-concentrated as the original grain. Furthermore, once it is milled, the grain loses its complexity. Examine flour closely and you will notice that the large grains of whole wheat have become small, very fine particles that look like dust. These particles are processed by the body much more rapidly than the complex whole grain.

If refined flour is twice as dense as whole wheat after the milling process, then the products made from that flour will also pack an additional caloric density. Examine any package of pasta, locate the serving size, and you will notice that two ounces of dry pasta contain 210 calories. Two ounces of dry pasta is less than a small handful! Grab a 210-calorie baked potato, and it will fill your hand.

Lotsa Pasta and Bigger Bagels

I conducted an experiment in one of my eating management workshops. I asked everybody to cook the amount of pasta they would normally eat. We made a low fat sauce to go with it. When everyone had prepared the dish, I weighed each bowl and showed them how many calories they would be eating. Everyone was shocked to discover that the average size bowl of pasta contained between 850 and 1,100 calories—before the sauce was added!

Because they are made from wheat gluten flour, which contains five hundred calories per cup, bagels are even more calorically dense than pasta. Moreover, because of their recent surge in popularity, larger bagels are being sold. Don't be surprised to discover that the bagels you have been feeding your child contain four hundred to five hundred calories. Often, bagels are a binge food. If your child is consuming two or three per day, the excessive intake of carbohydrates can slow down fat loss.

Most products made from processed flour fall under the same category as pasta and breads. No matter how low in fat they are, eating too many pretzels, crackers, bread sticks, and cereals can slow down weight loss.

The point is *not* that these foods are off limits, but too many of them can increase your child's total calories more than you may realize. Reduce the amount of processed flour your child consumes if he is having trouble dropping body fat. Replace these foods with lean meats and complex carbohydrates. A chicken breast and a small baked potato contain more nutritional value and fewer calories than an average size bagel. A piece of fish with steamed new potatoes (avoiding high fat condiments), will produce a much better weight loss than will eating a large bowl of pasta.

Complex Carbohydrates That May Cause Your Child to Gain Weight

Bagels	Flour-based foods	Pretzels
Crackers	Pasta	Too much bread

Fruits and Vegetables

No one would dispute that increasing vitamins and minerals by eating more fruits and vegetables is the best way to improve your child's health. Extensive research has demonstrated that fruits and vegetables may protect the human body from disease when eaten in sufficient quantities. Studies have shown that people who consume a lot of fruits and vegetables have lower rates of cancer, most likely because fruits and vegetables contain fiber, antioxidants such as beta-carotene and vitamin C, and chemical compounds called phytochemicals.

Fruits contain limonene, ellagic acid, ferulic acid, and caffeic acid, all of which help increase the production of enzymes that may help scavenge, dispose of, and prevent carcinogens (chemical compounds that promote cancer) from altering a cell's DNA. Cruciferous (green leafy) vegetables such as broccoli, bok choy, and brussels sprouts contain dithiolthiones, indoles, and isothiocyanates that trigger the formation of enzymes that help block carcinogens from damaging cells. Grains also contain a number of phytochemicals that may help slow down the reproduction of cells in the large intestine, thereby reducing the risk of colon cancer.

You don't need to memorize all these fancy words, but simply be aware that in addition to helping your child lose weight, fresh fruits and vegetables work to protect your child's body from disease.

Many parents find it easier and more convenient at first to increase their child's intake of fruit because most kids like fruit, and fruit doesn't need to be cooked—it can be carried "as is" and eaten just about anywhere.Use caution with non-organically grown fruits and vegetables, which may contain unwanted pesticides. Purchase fruits with thick skins that can be removed, such as bananas, oranges, pineapples, and watermelons, whose peels and rinds act as natural barriers to pesticides; and always wash fruit before serving.

Avoid canned fruit, because usually it is high in sugar. Fruit juices and dried fruits, though low in fat, contain a lot of calories and may interfere with a child's ability to lose weight. Here's a list of healthy fruits to feed your child:

Apples	Grapefruit	Passion fruit
Applesauce (unsweetened)	Grapes	Peaches
Apricots	Honeydew melon	Pears
Bananas	Kiwi	Pineapple
Blackberries	Mangoes	Plums
Blueberries	Nectarines	Raisins
Cantaloupe	Oranges	Raspberries
Cherries	Papayas	Strawberries
		Watermelon

There is no such thing as a bad vegetable—unless, of course, you fry it or convert it into a high fat snack like potato chips or carrot cake. Vegetables contain many significant vitamins and minerals, are low in fat, and often contain a lot of fiber. Fiber-rich foods, coupled with a high water intake, eliminate most bouts of constipation and reduce the risk of colon cancer. Fiber acts as tiny sponges within the intestines and absorbs many times its weight in water. As a result, the feces become softer and bulkier, making movement through the intestines easier.

Pick out vegetables that your child likes. If she only likes one or two, center your recipes around those. One sneaky but effective way to introduce vegetables is to add small quantities to other dishes. Your kids probably won't notice some added spinach in your lasagna because the fat-free cheese and tomato sauce will cover up its taste. A child who doesn't like tomatoes may love tomato sauce in other dishes. Try adding water chestnuts to a tuna sandwich. Steaming vegetables in chicken broth adds to their flavor. Here's a list of healthy vegetables to serve your child:

Artichokes	Eggplant	Peppers
Asparagus	Green beans	Radishes
Bamboo shoots	Greens	Shallots
Broccoli	Leeks	Spinach
Brussels sprouts	Lettuce	Sprouts
Cabbage	Mushrooms	Tomatoes
Carrots	Okra	Water chestnuts
Cauliflower	Onions	Zucchini
Celery		

Protein

Protein is necessary to build tissue, maintain muscle, repair the body, and increase the metabolic rate. Our bodies don't use the protein itself, but the amino acids contained in protein are what we require. Protein also plays a role in the body's manufacturing of hormones and antibodies. Because your daughter is growing, and because protein serves so many different purposes and is utilized so quickly, it is best to replenish it in small amounts throughout the day. It isn't necessary to be on a high-protein diet, but it is important to serve high quality, low fat sources of protein along with complex carbohydrates. Low fat proteins help to build a strong, healthy body.

Twenty different amino acids are required to build muscle. Of these twenty, almost half can be made within the body. These "home grown" amino acids are referred to as *nonessential amino acids,* because they can be made by the body and therefore it is not essential that we ingest them in our diet. *Essential amino acids* are those which cannot be manufactured in the body and therefore must be ingested through our diet.

When a protein source contains all of the essential amino acids, it is termed a *complete protein.* Complete proteins are derived from animal sources, such as fish, poultry, beef, eggs and dairy products.

If a protein lacks any of the essential amino acids, it is called an incomplete protein. Incomplete proteins can sustain life but they lack certain amino acids necessary to promote growth. Incomplete proteins come from plant products, such as corn, rice, and beans, and must be combined with other protein sources to compose a complete set of amino acids. If you think your child is getting all the protein she needs from a bowl of beans, guess again!

The USDA's food pyramid divides proteins into two groups. One group contains dairy products such as yogurt, milk, and cheese; and the other contains meats, poultry, fish, beans, eggs, and nuts. Unfortunately, as discussed earlier, these categories fail to distinguish "good" and "bad" sources of protein. It would make more sense to group proteins according to their nutritional value, thereby making a distinction between healthier, low fat protein sources and others that are high in fat, cholesterol, and sodium. What makes matters difficult is that choosing a "good" source is not always a cut and dried decision.

Take meat, for example, the most common source of protein in the United States. Although meat is an excellent protein source, it usually comes with a heavy price tag of cholesterol and saturated fat. One three-and-one-half ounce serving contains an average of ninety-five milligrams of cholesterol, regardless of whether it's beef, pork, chicken, turkey, or fish. (Shellfish contain even more cholesterol than the other meats listed.)

Many people believe that all poultry and fish are good sources of protein because they are low in fat and that beef and pork are always bad sources of protein because they are high in saturated fat. However, whether a selection is good or bad depends on the cut of meat you are eating. Eating chicken doesn't guarantee that you are eating low fat. Some cuts of poultry contain more fat than certain cuts of beef. Depending on how it is prepared, some fish is very high in fat and cholesterol. Therefore, it is important to choose your cuts of meat carefully when you are trying to help your child lose weight.

Poultry

You might be surprised to discover that skinless chicken thighs, drumsticks, and wings are not low fat choices. Believe it or not, a chicken thigh is 54 percent fat! In fact, the thigh contains more saturated fat and total fat than an extra-lean beef round steak or sirloin. Wings and drumsticks are also very high in fat, even if you remove the skin. The wing has more fat than the drumstick. Only the white pieces of chicken or turkey are truly low fat, and then only if you remove the skin before cooking.

Be extremely careful when buying ground chicken or turkey. Whether or not these products are low fat choices depends entirely upon which part of the bird is ground up. To be truly low fat, ground poultry must be made from 100 percent breast meat. Ground poultry breast contains about 10 percent fat, whereas ground poultry that contains other high fat portions of the bird can be as high as 54 percent fat. Always read the label and calculate the percentage of fat before buying any ground meat.

Beef

Have you ever noticed that the beef used in advertisements usually looks very lean? Because the beef industry wants to emphasize how lean red meat can be, they advertise the best, leanest cuts. Of course, the nutrition numbers and facts used in these ads reflect only the lower fat, select cuts of beef, which may be a whole lot different from the beef you purchase from your local butcher or grocery store.

But don't be discouraged. When it comes to red meat, there are Better Bad Choices. If you want to feed your child red meat, choose the leaner cuts, like top round, eye of round, tenderloin, and sirloin. If you shop at a full-service meat counter, ask the butcher to trim off all visible fat.

All cuts of veal contain between 35 percent and 50 percent fat, which makes veal a high fat food.

Pork, "The Other White Meat"

In an effort to position pork in the same favorable category as chicken and turkey, recent industry ads refer to pork as "the other white meat," implying that pork is as lean as white-meat poultry. Don't be fooled. Even though cooked pork is light in color, it is nowhere near as low in fat as chicken or turkey breast. The pork industry isn't playing fair when it uses the leanest cut (the tenderloin) for comparison, because less than 5 percent of all the pork sold in the United States comes from the tenderloin. In other words, 95 percent of the pork that Americans buy is higher fat cuts.

Luncheon Meats

Whatever you do, don't feed your child processed deli or luncheon meats. These meats are not what you think. Regardless of how fast, convenient, and easy to serve they are, don't touch these fabricated meats with a ten-foot cattle prod! It doesn't matter whether you buy all your luncheon meats at the service-deli counter or grab the nearest package from Oscar Mayer, all deli meats have been processed to extend their shelf life.

Years ago, the meat industry discovered that by using certain chemicals, binders, and fillers, they could reduce losses due to spoilage. In essence, they extended the shelf life of a meat from one week to three months and, in so doing, increased profits substantially.

Have you noticed that all deli meats have a completely different texture than meat sliced from a real turkey or chicken? Processing meats requires certain trade-offs, one of which is the need to add binders and fillers to give the meat the right mouth feel and consistency. But here's the catch: Binders and fillers leave less room for protein and other important nutrients. Consequently, most luncheon meats have a lower protein content than real meats.

I sent a turkey breast to a lab for chemical analysis. Eight ounces of turkey contained a mere 148 milligrams of sodium. I then sent a low fat turkey-breast luncheon meat to the same lab, and guess what? It contained an astounding 1647 milligrams of sodium! Worse yet, the sodium in deli meat isn't the same kind that occurs naturally in a real turkey. Deli meats contain sodium nitrite and sodium nitrate. Sodium nitrate is also known as saltpeter! Saltpeter alters the hormonal system in humans, which can decrease sex drive and cause weight gain. (It's also used in gunpowder.) Sodium nitrite is a known carcinogen, causing cancer in humans.

Carcinogens like sodium nitrite may take years to cause cancer; it won't happen from just one bite. But if you feed your child luncheon meats of any kind, they are much more likely to develop cancer later in life then a child who never eats processed meats. Another form of sodium used in luncheon meats (as well as baked goods and beverages) is sodium erythorbate, which is used to accelerate color fixing in the curing process. Even though sodium erythorbate is on the FDA's Generally-Regarded-As-Safe list, why eat it if you don't have to?

Fish

Some fish are very high in fat and should be avoided when you are trying to reduce your child's weight. Catfish, herring, mackerel, salmon, trout, swordfish, and eel contain between 25 percent and 50 percent fat! Choose low fat fish like cod, red snapper, flounder, bass, perch, pike, and fresh tuna. Shellfish, including shrimp, oysters, and lobster, are usually very high in cholesterol but low in saturated fat.

Canned varieties of fish are nutritionally inferior to their fresh counterparts. Avoid fish canned in oil, in favor of water-packed varieties. Some brands of albacore tuna become higher in fat at certain times of year. In addition, the sodium content of canned fish is often very high. Look for low sodium or reduced-sodium varieties, available in most stores.

Be wary of seafood that is displayed stacked high on ice. Although the fish may look attractive, food poisoning can occur if the seafood on top of the stack becomes too warm. Warmer temperatures allow bacteria to thrive. Bacteria that contaminate one stack of fish can move via air currents to other fish displayed around the contaminated batch. If the seafood is subsequently undercooked, or if you purchase contaminated seafood already cooked, your child could develop a severe case of food poisoning. Always buy fish from the bottom of the stack or as close to the ice as possible.

Dairy Products

Dairy products are exceptionally high-quality sources of protein and contain terrific balances of amino acids. With all the new brands of fat-free foods available—cheese, sour cream, cream cheese, cottage cheese, and milk—eating low fat has never been easier. Steer your child away from high fat dairy products, such as whole milk, regular cheese, and egg yolks, by substituting lower fat products like skim milk, low fat or fat-free cheeses, and low fat cottage cheese.

The only reason your child would need to avoid the dairy group is if she suffers from lactose intolerance. Lactose intolerance means that your child lacks the enzyme necessary to digest milk sugars. Symptoms include gas, bloating, diarrhea, and possibly skin rashes or eczema. However, there is a special milk called Lactaid, which contains lactase, the milk sugar digestive enzyme. Lactaid milk tastes great, and can be used just like regular milk by lactose-intolerant children.

Here's a list of healthy, low fat sources of protein to feed your child.

Low Fat Sources of Protein (under 20 percent fat)

Chicken breast	Imitation crab	Skim milk
Cod	Lobster	Snapper
Crab	Low fat cottage cheese	Sole
Egg whites	Low fat yogurt	Turkey breast
Fat-free cheeses	Ocean perch	
Flounder	Scallops	
Haddock	Shark	
Halibut	Shrimp	

Chapter 7

Pitfalls on the Road to Weight Control

Sugar

Some Not So Sweet Facts

Americans eat their weight in sugar each year. On average, this amounts to 140 pounds per person. Ouch! You may find this figure hard to believe if you don't add much sugar to the foods you eat, but most of the sugar we eat is added into our diet by the food industry. You may not be aware that sugar is hidden in the vast majority of processed foods. Sugar is often added to salad dressing, soup, tomato sauce, yogurt, and even processed meats. Sugar is hard to avoid, especially if your child eats canned or processed foods.

Regular soft drinks are a major culprit. A twelve-ounce can of soda contains up to thirteen teaspoons of sugar. Does your child have more than one soda per day? Drinking three regular sodas a day is the same as eating thirty-nine teaspoons of sugar. No parent would knowingly feed a child thirty-nine teaspoons of sugar in one day. Taking our example a step further, if your son drinks three regular sodas every day for a week, he will have consumed 273 teaspoons of sugar, or 95 tablespoons, which would add up to 308 *cups* of sugar in a year! If your son is drinking three regular sodas per day, simply switching him to diet soda would trim more than 600 empty calories *per day* from his diet.

What Does Sugar Have to Do with Fat?

Sugar consumption contributes to childhood obesity as much as high fat foods. Although sugar doesn't contain any fat, it is rapidly converted into body fat when your son eats more than his body can burn off. Although sugar is a carbohydrate, it contains virtually no vitamins or minerals. Worse yet, high-sugar foods tend to push more nutritious foods out of the diet.

In an effort to make their products appear healthier, some food manufacturers will tout their use of peach concentrate, pear concentrate, or other fruit sweeteners. Ignore the hype. Regardless of whether it is white sugar, brown sugar, corn syrup, rice syrup, glucose, fructose, molasses or honey, as far as your child's body is concerned, it's sugar.

Sugar also contributes to heart disease, because it is converted to triglycerides by the body—especially fructose, a processed sugar derived from fruit. Although not many ten-year-olds have advanced heart disease, we know that the seeds of this disease are planted at an early age. Children as young as six can show elevated triglyceride and cholesterol levels. Although it may take many years, by the time the effects of an unhealthy diet show, they may be too late to reverse. And let's not forget the role that excessive sugar intake can play in the development of diabetes.

Another concern is diabetes. Contrary to popular belief, eating too much sugar doesn't directly cause this disease. However, obesity caused by excess consumption can trigger diabetes. Diabetes in children has reached an all-time high, and this is not just due to genetics. Lifestyle decisions have a lot to do with it. If you child has a weight problem because you allow him to eat too many snacks or fast food, this is a lifestyle problem that can be reversed. Just altering the frequency with which your child indulges in these potentially harmful behaviors may prevent the onset of a life-threatening disease.

Tooth decay is another problem associated with excessive sugar consumption. Think of all the money you will save in dental bills simply by limiting the amount of sugar your child eats.

How Much Sugar Is Okay?

Product labels list the amount of sugar, in grams, that foods contain. Tally these numbers for one average day to see how many grams of sugar your daughter eats. If you can keep her daily sugar intake to below sixty grams, you deserve a pat on the back. If you keep it under forty grams, you're doing even better. Consumption of more than sixty grams of sugar a day is cause for concern.

The Sugar Formula

Although the United States has not converted to the metric system, our food labels list nutritional information in terms of grams. All labels, by law, must list the grams of sugar. A more familiar unit of measure for sugar is teaspoons. Fortunately, converting sugar from grams to teaspoons is easy. There are four grams to a teaspoon. Simply take the number of grams of sugar listed on a label and divide by four to calculate the number of teaspoons of sugar in one serving of that particular food. For example, a can of regular soda lists forty grams of sugar. Forty grams divided by four (40/4) is ten teaspoons of sugar. The sugar formula is short and sweet!

Choosing Low Sugar Cereals

Now that you know how to convert grams of sugar into teaspoons, choosing a good cereal for your child should be easy. But don't forget to consider the serving size listed on the package. If the serving size is one ounce, but your daughter consumes three ounces, she is eating three times as much sugar. If the cereal already contains sugar, don't let her dump more on top! The best way to avoid the habit of adding sugar is not to start in the first place. Remove the sugar bowl from the table. Out of sight, out of mind!

Nutrition Facts
Serving Size 1 can (360ml)

Amount Per Serving

Calories 140

	% Daily Value*
Total Fat 0g	0%
Sodium 20 mg	1%
Total Carbohydrate 36g	12%
Sugars 40gm	
Protein 0g	0%

*Percent Daily Values are based on a 2,000 caloric diet

In the appendix, I have listed the most popular breakfast cereals, along with how many grams and teaspoons of sugar are in each serving. The serving size is determined by the food manufacturers, but in most cases is about thirty grams of cereal. Depending on the density of the cereal, thirty grams amounts to anywhere from one-half cup to a full cup. I have also shown the percentage of sugar for each cereal, based on total calories. If the sugar listing for a cereal is 50 percent, it means half the cereal's calories come from sugar!

Eliminate Beverages That Contain Calories

One easy way to help your daughter lose weight is to eliminate beverages that contain calories from her diet. Regular sodas, milkshakes, juices, and some iced tea products contain so many calories from sugar that they may hamper your daughter's ability to lose weight.

The incredible variety of iced teas, sodas, flavored waters, and sports drinks on the market make it difficult to decide what your child should drink—especially when the marketers of these products go out of their way to make these drinks appear healthy. A quick glance at the number of grams of sugar will remove confusion about what's healthy and what's not.

Let's take a look at Snapple, a popular beverage. It appears this drink contains twenty-nine grams, or seven and one-fourth teaspoons, of sugar in one bottle. But when you look closely at the label, you will notice that the twenty-nine gram listing is *per serving*, not per bottle. Each bottle is advertised to contain two servings, which translates into fifty-eight grams of sugar per bottle. A full bottle of Snapple, which is marketed as a natural beverage, is the equivalent of a glass of water filled with fourteen and a half teaspoons of sugar. Always compare the listed serving size to the actual amount of the product that your child will consume.

Are Some Sugars More Natural Than Others?

White sugar, or sucrose, is derived from sugar cane or sugar beets, both of which grow naturally in the ground. Corn syrup and fruit sugar (fructose) also are made from natural products. However, once the corn, fruit, beet or cane is processed, the fiber, vitamins, minerals and water from the original plant are no longer present. Only the sweetness and the calories remain. No matter what the original source is, sugar is sugar, and it's time we started treating all sugars equally. Listed below are several popular beverages along with the number of calories and the approximate teaspoons of sugar contained in each.

Product	Calories per serving	Grams sugar	Teaspoons sugar
All Sport, 8 ounce	76	19	4 3/4
Apple Juice, 8 ounce	110	28	7
A&W Root Beer, 12 ounce	170	46	11 1/2
Big Red, 12 ounce	150	38	9 1/2
Calistoga Tea, 16 ounce	215	54	13 1/2
Capri Sun, pouch	100	27	6 3/4
Celestial Seasonings Tea, 16 ounce	164	41	10 1/4
Cherry Coke, 12 ounce	150	42	10 1/2
Clearly Canadian, 10 ounce	120	30	7 1/2
Coca-Cola, 12 ounce	140	39	9 3/4
Cranapple, 8 ounce	50	13	3 1/4
Dr. Pepper, 12 ounce	150	40	10
Frutopia, 16 ounce	220	60	15
Gatorade, 8 ounce	50	14	3 1/2
Grape Juice, 8 ounce	170	40	10
Grapefruit Juice, 8 ounce	120	28	7
Hawaiian Punch, 8 ounce	120	29	7 1/4
Ice Mountain, 11 ounce	119	30	7 1/2

Product	Calories per serving	Grams sugar	Teaspoons sugar
Kool Aid Bursts	100	24	6
Mistic Waters, 11 ounce	120	30	7 1/2
Mondo Fruit Squeeze	130	31	7 3/4
Mountain Dew, 12 ounce	170	46	11 1/2
Nestea, 16 ounce	176	44	11
Orange Juice, 8 ounce	120	28	7
Poweraid	70	15	3 3/4
Pepsi, 12 ounce	150	41	10 1/4
RC Cola, 12 ounce	165	43	10 3/4
7-Up, 12 ounce	140	39	9 3/4
Sprite, 8 ounce	150	39	9 3/4
Slice Orange Soda, 12 ounce	190	50	12 1/2
Slice Red Soda, 12 ounce	190	50	12 1/2
Snapple Tea, 16 ounce	200	50	12 1/2
Squirt, 12 ounce	150	40	10
Sundance, 10 ounce	120	30	7 1/2
Sunny Delight, 8 ounce	120	27	6 3/4
Tang, 8 ounce	150	34	8 1/2
V-8 Juice, 11 ounce	70	11	2 3/4
Welch's Fruit Punch, 12 ounce	190	51	12 3/4
Welch's Grape Soda, 12 ounce	190	51	12 3/4
Welch's Strawberry Soda, 12 ounce	190	51	12 3/4

Most of these beverages are available in a diet version, which is a great alternative. If your son's favorite beverage comes in a diet version, I suggest switching.

Celestial Seasonings makes diet beverages that contain as few as four or eight calories; Snapple makes a diet version that contains only four calories; and Nestea makes a diet lemon tea that contains only sixteen calories. You may be surprised by how similar to the regular beverages these reduced-calorie drinks taste.

Five Quick Ways to Reduce Your Child's Sugar Intake
1. Read labels!

    Notice how many grams of sugar your son's food and beverages contain and try to keep the total number as low as possible. Switch from fruit juices, sodas, and other high sugar drinks to lower sugar alternatives, like diet sodas.

2. Beware of sugar wearing a disguise.

   Glucose, sucrose, dextrose, fructose, corn syrup, rice syrup, peach concentrate, molasses, honey, and brown sugar are all forms of sugar. The total amount of sugar in a product will always be listed on the Nutrition Facts label under Sugar. Divide the number of grams by four to determine how many teaspoons of sugar are in the product.

3. Reduce consumption of sugar-laden snacks.

   Cut down on the amount of pastries, cookies, candy, ice cream, and soft drinks that your son consumes. Substitute fresh fruit and low-calorie desserts. Switch to diet versions such as NutraSweet Jell-O Pudding.

4. Choose a low-sugar cereal.

   Try to find at least three low-sugar cereals that your daughter likes. Keep them stocked in your pantry and rotate them to prevent boredom. Oatmeal, unfrosted Shredded Wheat, and Cheerios are excellent choices.

5. Reduce the amount of sugar you use in recipes.

   If a recipe calls for one cup of sugar, simply reduce it to three-quarters of a cup. Your children will never know the difference. As time goes on, reduce it even further. Eventually, you may find that you can cut back to a half a cup, with no change in taste. To help you get started, I've included in the recipes section a substitution list for modifying recipes.

Caffeine

Did you know that your kids may be consuming more caffeine than you are? If your son is fidgety, inattentive, easily distracted, impulsive, and unruly, it may be due to excessive caffeine consumption rather than attention deficit disorder (ADD). Because the symptoms of a high caffeine intake in children mimic the symptoms of attention deficit/hyperactivity disorder, it's easy to see how teachers and clinicians could mistakenly believe that a restless child has ADD. If your son has been diagnosed with ADD, try removing caffeine from his diet before using Ritalin.

One study checked the caffeine consumption of four hundred New York preschoolers, whose average age was four. It was discovered that almost 10 percent were ingesting at least two and a half milligrams of caffeine per pound of body weight (equal to about two cups of coffee for a 150-pound adult). Four percent of the children were found to be consuming the equivalent of at least three cups of coffee a day. A twelve ounce can of soda plus a half cup of freshly brewed iced tea contains as much caffeine as three cups of coffee.

Caffeine Is a Drug

Caffeine is part of a group of compounds, called methylxanthines, that occur naturally in many different plant products, including coffee beans, tea leaves, cocoa beans, and kola nuts. Most adults consume caffeine in coffee, but sodas are the number one source of caffeine consumed by children. Americans consume almost one-fifth of the world's 6.5-million-ton coffee production. Coffee contains more than 393 chemicals, and one cup contains anywhere from 40 to 170 milligrams of caffeine.

Caffeine is unquestionably a drug. Millions of people can attest to the withdrawal symptoms they experience whenever they try to give it up. Like most drugs, the more caffeine your child consumes, the greater his tolerance becomes to the negative aspects. Caffeine acts as a stimulant by working directly on the central nervous system, thereby increasing energy levels, alertness, and mental focus. It is absorbed very rapidly in your child's system and reaches peak concentrations about one hour after ingestion.

Caffeine can cause a number of side effects, depending on how much your child consumes and how high his tolerance is. It can cause his blood pressure to soar, increase his heart rate, potentially cause sleeplessness, and act as a diuretic. If your son's tolerance is low, he may experience irritability, headaches, trembling, nervousness, and bedwetting, many of the same symptoms that indicate attention deficit disorder.

What Products Contain Caffeine, and How Much?

The table shows the approximate caffeine content of some foods and beverages.

Item	Caffeine, mg (average)	Caffeine, mg (range)
Coffee, 5 ounce cup		
Brewed, drip method	115	60–180
Brewed, percolator	80	40–170
Instant	65	30–120
Decaffeinated, brewed	3	2–5
Decaffeinated, instant	2	1–5
Tea, 5 ounce cup		
Brewed, major U.S. brands	40	20–90
Brewed, imported brands	60	25–119
Instant	30	25–50
Iced tea, 12 ounce glass	70	67–76
Some soft drinks, 12 ounce	36	30–60
Cocoa beverage, 10 ounce	8	4–40

Item	Caffeine, mg (average)	Caffeine, mg (range)
Chocolate milk beverage, 8 ounce	5	2–7
Milk chocolate, 1 ounce	6	1–15
Dark chocolate, semi-sweet, 1 ounce	20	5–35
Baker's chocolate, 1 ounce	26	26
Chocolate-flavored syrup, 1 ounce	4	4

What Else Should You Know about Caffeine?

Caffeine may also cause problems by interacting with medications. Some drugs hamper a body's ability to excrete caffeine, which means that even small amounts of coffee can cause insomnia, irritability, and heart palpitations. Some stimulants may exhibit increased potency when taken in combination with a few cups of coffee a day. Asthma drugs, appetite suppressants, and thyroid medications may increase the jolt from caffeine. If your child suffers from asthma or is taking any medications, ask your doctor about potential interactions. Caffeine can also wreak havoc on your son's blood sugar level and may aggravate hypoglycemia (low blood sugar).

The Straight Scoop on Caffeine

If your child regularly consumes large amounts of caffeine, it could cause behavioral changes and health problems. Find other beverages for your child that don't contain caffeine. Possible alternatives include Crystal Light, NutraSweetened Kool-Aid, water, or a small amount of juice diluted with club soda.

Is Aspartame Bad for My Child?

Aspartame is made from two amino acids, phenylalanine and aspartic acid. Like all amino acids, these two are found abundantly in every high-protein food your child eats. When these two amino acids are joined together, they create a compound that tastes like sugar, but is two hundred times sweeter than normal sugar. Aspartame contains the same four calories per gram as all other sugars, but because it is so sweet, only a tiny amount is required to sweeten foods. Aspartame is used in just about every kind of food imaginable, including fat-free sweets, reduced-calorie ice creams, cookies, and diet sodas. Two well-known brands of aspartame powder are Equal and NutraSweet.

But I Heard Aspartame Is Bad!

Critics focus on the way aspartame breaks down in the body and claim it causes all kinds of health problems. When aspartame is ingested or heated, it breaks down and converts into methanol. After being converted into methanol, it is converted to formaldehyde, which in turn converts to formic acid. Formic acid is a known carcinogen, which is the source of the controversy and fear. Many foods that do not contain aspartame, including certain fruits and vegetables, go through a similar breakdown.

Researchers set out to determine whether levels of methanol and formaldehyde were increased in the bloodstream of aspartame users and whether any discernible differences could be detected between users and nonusers. Scientists at Harvard Medical School, the University of Arizona College of Medicine, and the University of Michigan School of Public Health concluded that:

(a) There were no differences in blood levels of methanol or formaldehyde in aspartame users versus nonusers.

(b) There were no links to seizures or hyperactivity, although a harmless elevation of the amino acid phenylalanine was observed in the bloodstream after subjects were fed very high dosages of aspartame.

So Who Should Avoid Aspartame?

The following four groups should stay away from aspartame:
1. Children who are allergic to aspartame;
2. Children who have phenylketonuria;
3. Pregnant women, and women who are breast-feeding;
4. Those who for philosophical reasons want to avoid it.

1. *Children who are allergic to aspartame.* As with all foods, chemicals, and substances, some children have a food sensitivity and/or allergic reaction to aspartame. These problems are no different than if a child were sensitive to tomatoes, milk, seafood, or any other food. As with any food sensitivity, the degree of symptoms varies. Because some people are allergic, some health enthusiasts advocate that everyone should avoid aspartame. But if someone had an allergy to tomatoes or milk, would we issue an alert telling everyone to avoid tomatoes and milk? Of course not.

2. *Children who have phenylketonuria.* Another group that should avoid aspartame are those who suffer from a syndrome called phenylketonuria (PKU). PKU prevents a child from properly metabolizing the amino acid phenylalanine. Children who suffer from this disorder develop extremely high levels of phenylalanine in their bloodstreams, which may lead to brain damage. PKU occurs at birth and is usually diagnosed very early in life. Two percent of the U.S. population, about 4.5 million people, have one of the two genes necessary for PKU. Although critics of aspartame contend that these individuals may be sensitive to phenylalanine, possessing one gene does not make a person susceptible to the same reactions seen with PKU. A child must have both genes to develop problems

metabolizing phenylalanine. It's not that children with PKU cannot eat aspartame, it's that it needs to be added to their daily allotment of phenylalanine.

3. *Pregnant women, and women who are breast-feeding.* The topic of whether pregnant and breast-feeding women should avoid aspartame is hotly debated. While some doctors believe there is no problem with its use, others advise any pregnant woman to avoid aspartame because of the possible risk that her fetus possesses both genes that cause PKU. Because the risk does exist, I encourage pregnant women to avoid aspartame.

4. *Those who for philosophical reasons want to avoid it.* Some people believe that anything that doesn't occur naturally is bad. If you agree, then you should certainly omit aspartame from your child's diet.

The Health Food Store Contradiction

Aspartame is not universally regarded as completely safe, but there are inconsistencies in the food industry. For example, some health food stores boycott aspartame because they believe that high concentrations of phenylalanine are dangerous and toxic, yet they sell phenylalanine as an amino acid supplement in dosages of five hundred milligrams per tablet! The dosage in one five hundred milligram tablet contains more phenylalanine than twenty-seven packets of Equal. If a five hundred milligram dose of phenylalanine is considered safe as a dietary supplement, why would eighteen milligrams—the amount in one package of Equal—be harmful?

Fake Fats

Fat Substitutes

As concern about health and nutrition has increased, manufacturers have scrambled to produce as many low fat and fat-free foods as possible.

Because most consumers don't want to give up their favorite high fat foods in favor of foods naturally low in fat, manufacturers have responded by finding ways to produce their top-selling high fat products with the fat removed or replaced. The solution has been the creation of a new breed of calorie- and fat-reduction agents that now account for more than 30 percent of the four-billion-dollar food additives market.

No fat replacement is entirely versatile. Most cannot withstand changes in temperature without altering some of their properties. Unlike normal fats, you cannot heat, freeze, or fry fat substitutes, or store them at room temperature.

Replacing all the attributes of fat is very complicated because fat has physical properties such as texture, lubricity, viscosity, and structural stability that contribute to the overall texture, appearance, and flavor of the product. Fat is not a single compound. It's a family of fatty acids, with saturated or unsaturated chains consisting of between eight and eighteen carbons. Depending on the combination of chain lengths and the degree of saturation, fats will possess very different physical properties, which is what allows natural fat to accommodate very different uses. Depending on its chemical structure and how it is processed, a fat substitute can be manipulated to mimic some but not all fat properties.

Fat substitutes are divided into three categories:
- Carbohydrate-based substitutes
- Protein-based substitutes
- Fat-based substitutes

Carbohydrate-Based Fat Substitutes

These are the safest form of fat substitute for your child. Carbohydrates (or starches) contain four calories per gram, whereas fat contains nine calories per gram. When mixed with water to form bland gels, starches can mimic the bulk and texture of fat. Because water is the primary ingredient, the number of calories can be reduced to one calorie per gram or less. In fact, these substitutes often can replace up to 100 percent of the fat in many foods. Examples of carbohydrate-based fat substitutes are modified food starches such as polydextrose, cellulose, dextrin, maltodextrin, and various gums such as xanthan, locust bean, guar, and carrageenan.

Carbohydrate-based substitutes are usually sold as powders, which have a longer shelf life and are easier to handle than premixed gels. When the mixture is heated, stirred, and cooled, it stabilizes water into a heat-stable, jelled, fat-like structure that can be used in baking. These products cannot be used in frying, however, because they melt and disintegrate at high temperatures. The gel-like product that results after mixing the powder with water is gum. You may have noticed these gums mentioned as ingredients on product labels.

Some manufacturers have begun to establish brand identities for their fat substitutes. An example of a carbohydrate-based product is Oatrim (also called LEANesse). Derived from an enzymatic treatment of oat flour and oat bran, Oatrim gives foods a creamier taste and texture than other fat replacements and is often used in salad dressings, baked goods, and ice cream. ConAgra's Healthy Choice extra lean ground beef also is made using Oatrim. Compared to a supermarket's extra lean ground beef, which contains about 270 calories and twenty grams of fat, the same serving size of Healthy Choice beef contains 130 calories and four grams of fat.

Protein-Based Fat Substitutes

Simplesse, made by the NutraSweet company, is the only protein-based fat replacement available in the United States. Made from egg-white protein or milk protein and sold in either liquid or powder form, Simplesse is used in everything from cheese and ice cream to salad dressing and mayonnaise. Because proteins break down when exposed to heat, most protein-based substitutes can only be used in cold food products and a few baked goods. They cannot be used for frying.

Protein-based substitutes are designed to mimic the lubricity of fats by using protein broken down into very small particles. These tiny particles are perceived in the mouth as creamy. Like carbohydrates, proteins contain four calories per gram, but fat replacements derived from protein contain only two calories per gram.

Fat-Based Fat Substitutes

It may appear contradictory to make a fat substitute from fat, but it is possible to create chemically altered fatty acids that contain few or no calories. By altering the size, shape, or structure of fat-like molecules, products have been developed that possess most or all of the characteristics of normal fats, but which are not metabolized by the body. Procter & Gamble introduced Olestra, a fat-based substitute derived from vegetable oils, that can be used in frying.

Due to its unique properties, Olestra possesses all of the characteristics of normal fats. Procter & Gamble claims that Olestra passes through the digestive tract unchanged and unabsorbed. Because Olestra is a bigger fat molecule, it is not hydrolyzed by digestive enzymes. Theoretically, you could fry potatoes, eat them, and only receive the calories from the potato. Procter & Gamble now uses Olestra in some of its potato, tortilla and corn chips.

The Center for Science in the Public Interest tried to block the FDA from allowing Olestra onto the market, insisting that it needs more testing. Studies have shown that Olestra blocks the absorption of many fat-soluble vitamins, such as A, D, E, and K. Instead, they get trapped with the Olestra and end up being eliminated rather than reaching the bloodstream.

Procter & Gamble admits that Olestra attaches to fat-soluble vitamins. To compensate, they fortify the chips with additional fat-soluble vitamins. Olestra has caused diarrhea in many test subjects. Any fat substitute that causes diarrhea and hasn't been widely tested should be used with caution. My advice is that you should limit the amount of Olestra that your children eat until longer-term studies have been conducted. However, chips made from this substitute do contain less fat and calories. In essence—a Better Bad Choice.

Fat-based substitutes showed great promise when first developed. However, they have lost some of their appeal because of the success and safety of carbohydrate-based substitutes. To date, very few fat-based substitutes have gained approval from the FDA and their future doesn't look bright.

The New Food Labels

In 1994, through a joint effort of the Food and Drug Administration (FDA) and the USDA, a nutrition labeling law went into effect for all packaged foods. In addition to requiring product labels to include specific nutritional information, the law attempted to set a standard to be followed before a product can be marketed as "light" or "lite." Voluntary programs for many raw foods such as fruits, vegetables, fish, and meats also were established.

These food labels were intended to offer more complete, useful, and accurate information than ever before. Unfortunately, companies found ways to get around the new label laws, and some have resorted to misleading marketing tactics. Some products that are marketed as "reduced fat" are not as low in fat as they appear. And even though a product contains less fat, it may not be a Better Bad Choice if it contains more calories and sugar. With all the fat-free and reduced-fat products popping up, it's easy to lose sight of total calories, sugar content, and serving sizes.

Misleading Labels

If a Label Claims That a Product Has Less Fat, It's Not Necessarily a Low Fat Food!

Like a good magician who waves one arm to distract your attention, many companies make alluring claims to trick you into purchasing their lower fat versions. For example, a box of Reduced Fat Triscuits claims that the product contains 40 percent less fat than regular Triscuits. But what Nabisco doesn't tell you is that this comparison is based upon measuring fat *by weight*, not fat by calories. It would be easy to assume that 40 percent less fat means 40 percent fewer calories, but that conclusion is incorrect. Yes, three grams of fat is 40 percent less than five grams of fat, but that number doesn't consider the calories. Using our fat formula to determine the percentage of fat reveals that the two types of Triscuits actually differ by a mere 11 percent fat. This practice is commonly used with crackers, ice cream, microwave popcorn, and cookies.

What about Foods That Are Labeled "Light" or "Reduced Fat"?

Don't fall prey to the deceptive word "light" on a label. Unfortunately, the new laws have not done away with many of these vague terms. "Light" is used to describe any food whose fat content has been reduced by 50 percent or its calories reduced by 33 percent from the original product. But "light" doesn't mean the product is necessarily low in fat or calories.

The term "reduced fat" can be equally deceiving. By law, "reduced fat" means that the food has 25 percent less fat than the same brand's regular product. But a reduced-fat version of a super-premium ice cream may still contain twelve grams of fat in a half-cup serving. Twelve grams *is* 25 percent less fat than the sixteen grams found in the regular product, but twelve grams of fat is still more fat than many regular ice creams contain.

Don't Forget to Compare Serving Sizes

Another way that a company can mislead you is by comparing different serving sizes. Pick up a bag of regular Fig Newtons and compare it to a bag of fat-free Fig Newtons. Although the serving size for both is the same number of cookies, you might easily overlook the fact that what is being compared is a thirty-one gram portion with a twenty-nine gram portion, which makes it difficult for the consumer to compare apples with apples, or in this case figs with figs. When you adjust the serving size of the regular Fig Newtons to equal the fat-free Fig Newtons, you'll find that the calories between the two products are almost identical.

Another practice is to charge more for the reduced-fat product. Almost all reduced-fat products cost the consumer more than the original counterpart, not because the reduced-fat products cost more to manufacture, but because the manufacturers have discovered that consumers are willing to pay extra when they see the words "fat-free," "reduced fat," or "light." Sometimes the price difference is concealed by differing package sizes. To continue our example from above, a package of fat-free Fig Newtons costs the same amount as a package of regular Fig Newtons— $3.19 at my local grocer. But even though the price is the same, the package of regular Fig Newtons contains sixteen ounces while the package of fat-free cookies contains only twelve ounces. Compared ounce for ounce, the fat-free Fig Newtons cost more. Such a deal!

Calories Do Matter

Did you know that many lower fat versions contain more sugar than the regular product? Sugar creates a pleasurable mouth feel, taste, and texture, which is why a product may still taste good even though fat has been removed. Sugar isn't as calorie-dense as fat, so you might think that the reduced-fat product should have fewer calories. Unfortunately, in many cases, it doesn't work that way. Food manufacturers understand that we want our favorite foods, only without the fat. In order to pass taste tests with their fat-free foods, many companies are compelled to use more sugar. Often, so much sugar is added that the calories in the fat-free foods equal or exceed the calories in the higher fat versions.

Don't forget calories when selecting lower fat products, and don't make the mistake of letting your child eat larger quantities of the lower fat food. An ounce of pretzels contains 110 calories, and an ounce of potato chips contains 140 calories—a difference of thirty calories per ounce. But the calorie savings will be obliterated if you replace one bag of chips eaten per week with two bags of pretzels. Choose the lower fat foods but keep your child's portion size the same or less if you want her to be able to lose weight.

When selecting Better Bad Choices for your child, make accurate comparisons. Compare serving sizes, ingredients, nutritional statements, and costs. You cannot rely solely on the fat or sugar listing.

Don't fall into the trap of buying additional quantities of a product simply because it is a Better Bad Choice. Let's face it: If a product is on your pantry shelf, it will be eaten. Watch out! One good way to limit your child's consumption of high fat products *and* too many Better Bad Choices is to buy only what you intend to eat each week. Develop your plan and stick to it.

Fat-Free Cooking Oil?

If you enjoy a good mystery, check out the nutritional information on a can of cooking spray the next time you go to the grocery store. Ingredients are always listed in descending order from most to least. The first ingredient listed on the cooking spray label is oil. Because the only other ingredients listed are propellants and water, we can surmise that the cooking spray is 100 percent fat.

Now look at the Nutrition Facts itemized on the label: zero grams of fat, zero calories from fat, and zero calories. No, you are not imagining things.

The loophole is based on the serving size, which in this case is listed as one-third of a second of spray. Get real. No one holds down the button for one-third of a second. The average spray time is probably more like two to three seconds. When I tested a can of cooking spray, it took about eight seconds to get a tablespoon of oil. A tablespoon of oil contains 120 calories and thirteen grams of fat, which means that two seconds of spray would contain approximately thirty calories and more than three grams of fat.

Even a one-third-of-a-second portion contains half a gram of fat, but the law allows a product that contains one-half gram of fat or less *per serving* to be labeled as "fat-free." By claiming a dubious one-third-of-a-second serving size, in this case a food that is 100 percent fat can claim to contain no fat.

Don't misunderstand. You can and should use these cooking sprays whenever you cook, because you can use less oil by spraying than by pouring. Nevertheless, be aware that "legal" product labels can be very deceptive and use cooking spray sparingly.

The Word "Lean" Doesn't Mean Low Fat

Beware of products that are labeled "lean." If your body were 45 percent fat, we wouldn't label you as lean. Yet according to the label laws, any meat that contains fewer than ten grams of fat per serving can be labeled lean. A lot of high fat meats have fewer than ten grams of fat per three ounce serving, but by no means are they low fat foods.

To make matters worse, ground meats are exempt from the new definitions. Consequently, "lean" or "extra lean" meats may be very high in fat. A popular package of "lean" ground turkey, labeled 7 percent fat (by weight), is actually 44 percent fat by calories (a very high fat food).

The legal definition of consumer fraud is "the deliberate intent to deceive one for the financial gain of another." Although many labels appear to fit the definition of consumer fraud, they may conform to USDA rules.

On the back label of a popular brand of ground turkey product, you will discover the Calories from Fat item. In this example, total calories are 160 and calories from fat are 70. If we divide fat calories by total calories we quickly determine that this ground turkey contains 44 percent fat—a far cry from the 7 percent fat claimed on the front label.

Another product claims to be 97 percent fat-free and contains less than one gram of fat per portion. It appears to be a low fat product, right? Would you be surprised to learn that this ham actually contains 29 percent fat when considering total calories? If we are trying to keep most of the foods we eat under 20 percent fat, this is not a low fat choice.

When you evaluate the claims on a product label, consider the portion size and evaluate the percentage of fat based on total calories, not percentage of fat by weight.

You might be able to make two or three sandwiches from this six ounce package of ham. But if you look at the "portions per container" listed on the label, you'll see that the manufacturer claims that the package contains fourteen to sixteen servings. Fourteen servings from a six ounce package of sliced meat is equivalent to putting a single potato chip on a slice of bread and calling it a sandwich!

This meat producer, as do many others, bases its assertion that its ham is "97 percent fat-free" on the percentage of fat in the product *by weight,* not by calories. When you consider that fat packs more than twice as many calories per gram of weight than either protein or carbohydrate, and when you factor in the percentage of the product's weight that comes from water, you can see that claiming 3 percent fat by weight disguises the truth that 29 percent of the product's calories come from fat.

Here's another way to understand the difference between percentage of fat by calories versus by weight. If you have a glass filled with half oil and half water, the half that is water is completely fat free. The half that is oil contains all the calories and every single calorie is from fat. If you drink the contents of the glass (assuming you could swallow it), 100 percent of the calories you consume will be from fat. Because all the calories within the glass come from fat, the glass should be labeled 100 percent fat. Of course, a marketing company would never label a product "100 percent fat," because they know you wouldn't buy it. Instead, they label the product by weight. Because half of the liquid is water, and water contains no fat, they would claim that the product is "50 percent fat-free."

I could show you example after example of how the food industry takes advantage of the labeling laws, but my purpose is to get *you* to look more closely and shop more carefully. The health of your family is at stake.

The Latest Buzzword

When researchers first reported that fiber reduces a person's risk of colon cancer, cereal companies scrambled to plaster "high fiber" in bold letters across their boxes. When it was announced that cholesterol contributes to heart disease, "cholesterol free" appeared on almost every product—from margarine to cookies. A high-fiber, low-cholesterol diet is good for you, but what appears on the label may not accurately represent what ends up in the box! Multi-grain waffles, bran muffins, and whole-wheat crackers may not contain as much bran or whole wheat as you think.

Remember, ingredients are listed according to how much of each went into the recipe. If a bread or cracker doesn't list "whole wheat" as the first ingredient, it's composed mostly of something else—probably white flour. According to the new label laws, any bread that uses the term "whole wheat" in its name must be made from 100 percent whole wheat flour. But the new laws say nothing about crackers, waffles, or muffins. A lot of breads, crackers, waffles, and muffins use terms such as "seven grain," "nutty grain," "multi-grain," or "made with oat bran" to give the perception that they are healthier to eat. Unfortunately, most of these products contain very little whole grain and a lot of white flour.

Weight Control for a Young America Recipes

Introduction

Let's suppose that you have a very finicky child. Every time you give your child turnips, she cries, has a tantrum, and closes her mouth as tight as a Federal Reserve Bank vault. Most parents don't understand that they give their child too many bribes and too many choices.

Here's a typical scenario: To get your child to quiet down at 3 P.M., you give your child a bunch of Doritos. Dinner is served at 5 P.M., and you wonder why your child won't eat. This sort of preemptive feeding is usually at the root of finicky eating.

First, the most important thing about feeding your children is giving them a *few* select choices. A couple of days per week, ask your child to choose dinner. Don't get into the habit of doing this every night, but regularly let your child choose something she wants. Be sure to present it in such a way that she has to choose between two healthy choices.

"Would you like to have turkey burgers with yam chips tonight or would you like lasagna?" Your child will feel good about making a choice and will be more inclined to eat dinner because she made the choice.

Second, whatever you cook for dinner is what your family will be eating. If your child refuses to eat, send her away from the table after dinner without eating. Don't worry about her starving. She will soon learn that if she doesn't eat what you fixed, she won't get anything. If she chooses not to eat what you cooked, do not let her have dessert or snack after dinner. Send her to bed hungry. Your child will learn very quickly that to get what she wants, she has to do what you want. <u>Don't budge on this point, ever!</u>

The best way to begin is to choose a recipe you think the whole family will like. Then, feel comfortable adding or subtracting items within the recipe. If your child doesn't like turnips, drop them and add something like carrots. Do this whenever you feel that substitution is appropriate. And don't forget that it's all right to substitute chicken breast for shrimp or vice versa.

Breakfast

Strawberry Oatmeal

1 ounce oatmeal cooked with water
2 tablespoons low sugar strawberry jam
3 sliced fresh strawberries

Make oatmeal according to directions using water. After oatmeal is cooked, stir in the strawberry jam until well blended. Slice fresh strawberries over oatmeal and serve.

Calories: 175 / Cholesterol: 0 / Protein: 2 grams / Fat: 1 gram / Fat: 6%

Blueberry Grits

1 ounce cooked grits
2 tablespoons low sugar blueberry preserves
1/2 cup fresh blueberries

Make grits according to directions using water. After grits are cooked, stir in blueberry preserves until well blended. Add fresh berries over grits and serve.

Calories: 220 / Cholesterol: 0 / Protein: 1 gram / Fat: 0 / Fat: 0

Cinnamon Raisin Oatmeal

1 ounce cooked oatmeal with water
2 tablespoons raisins
dash cinnamon

Cook oatmeal according to directions with water. Add raisins and sprinkle in cinnamon.

Calories: 160 / Cholesterol: 0 / Protein: 2 grams / Fat: 1 gram / Fat: 6%

Cheese Toast

2 slices lite whole wheat bread
2 slices low fat or fat-free cheese

Toast bread in toaster. While bread is toasting, turn on oven to broil. After toast is toasted, place a slice of cheese over each piece of toast and place on a cookie tray under the broiler for 1 to 2 minutes. Serve with a bowl of fresh fruit or slice of melon.

Calories: 170 / Cholesterol: 0 / Protein: 8 grams / Fat: 0 / Fat: 0

Dolce Bread

1 whole wheat English muffin
2 to 3 tablespoons fat-free cream cheese
2 to 3 tablespoons low sugar preserves, any flavor.
3/4 cup fresh fruit

Split English muffin in half and toast. Spread the cream cheese over both halves then coat with low sugar preserves. Serve with the bowl of fresh fruit.

Calories: 330 / Cholesterol: 0 / Protein: 4 grams / Fat: 1 gram / Fat: 3%

Yogurt Delight

4 sliced strawberries
1/2 diced orange
4 seedless grapes
1/4 diced apple
4 tablespoons nonfat plain yogurt
1 package Equal

Place all fruit in a large bowl, stir in yogurt and sprinkle in Equal. Serve.

Calories: 135 / Cholesterol: 0 / Protein: 3 grams / Fat: 0 / Fat: 0

Yogurt and Cereal

1 carton lite, low fat yogurt, any flavor
1 to 2 ounces high fiber, low sugar cereal (try Shredded Wheat or Grape Nuts)

Place cereal in a bowl. Stir yogurt until well blended and pour the yogurt over the cereal.

Calories: 200 / Cholesterol: 9 milligrams / Protein: 12 grams / Fat: 0 / Fat: 0

Potato Pancakes

1 cup dehydrated potato flakes
1/2 cup skim milk
3 raw egg whites or 1/4 cup Egg Beaters
2 tablespoons onion bits
1/2 teaspoon garlic salt
1/4 cup diced scallions or to taste
2 tablespoons pancake mix

Mix potato flakes with skim milk and egg whites. Stir in onion bits, garlic salt, scallions and pancake mix and stir well. If mix appears too dry, add more skim milk. Preheat skillet over medium heat with butter flavored cooking spray. Place heaping tablespoons of mix onto skillet. Cook until lightly brown, flip and cook until other side is golden brown. Serves 3.

Calories: 80 / Cholesterol: 2 milligrams / Protein: 6 grams / Fat: 0 / Fat: 0

Applesauce and Raisin Oatmeal

1 ounce oatmeal cooked with water
1/2 cup low sugar applesauce
2 tablespoons raisins
Dash cinnamon

Stir applesauce into oatmeal. Stir in cinnamon and raisins.

Calories: 210 / Cholesterol: 0 / Protein: 2 grams / Fat: 2 grams / Fat: 8%

French Toast

2 slices lite whole wheat bread
3 egg whites
2 tablespoons skim milk
1 teaspoon cinnamon
2 tablespoons lite maple syrup
Dash powdered sugar

Preheat a Teflon pan with butter flavored cooking spray over medium heat. Mix together egg whites cinnamon and skim milk. Dip bread in egg white mixture and place each slice in Teflon pan. Let each side brown. Place French toast on plate and lightly coat with syrup. Sprinkle with powdered sugar and serve.

Calories: 243 / Cholesterol: 0 / Protein: 14 grams / Fat: 1 gram / Fat: 4%

Bean and Cheese Burrito

2 egg whites
1/4 cup black beans
1 slice fat-free cheese
2 tablespoons diced onion
2 corn tortillas
2 tablespoons salsa
Dash chili powder and garlic powder

Scramble egg whites with beans, onion, salsa, chili and garlic powder. Place mixture in corn tortillas, add cheese, wrap and serve.

Calories: 220 / Cholesterol: 0 / Protein: 18 grams / Fat: 0 / Fat: 0

Fruit Flavored Pancake

3 raw egg whites
1/4 cup uncooked oatmeal
3 tablespoons any flavored low sugar preserves
2 tablespoons additional preserves

Place all the ingredients in a blender and mix on low. Spray a Teflon pan with butter flavored cooking spray and Preheat over medium heat. Pour mixture into Teflon pan and let cook until slightly firm. Turn cake over, let cook another 3 to 5 minutes. Remove from heat and spread additional preserves over pancake and serve.
By using blueberry preserves you will make blueberry pancakes. You can also use strawberry, raspberry, etc.

Calories: 210 / Cholesterol: 0 / Protein: 14 grams / Fat: 1 gram / Fat: 4%

Apple Cinnamon Raisin Pancake

3 raw egg whites
1/4 cup uncooked oatmeal
1/2 cup low sugar applesauce
3 tablespoons raisins
Dash cinnamon
3 tablespoons additional applesauce

Place all the ingredients in a blender and mix on low. Spray a Teflon pan with butter flavored cooking spray and preheat over medium heat. Pour mixture into Teflon pan and let cook until slightly firm. Turn cake over, let cook another 3 to 5 minutes. Remove from heat and spread additional applesauce over pancake and serve.

Calories: 225 / Cholesterol: 0 / Protein: 14 grams / Fat: 1 gram / Fat: 4%

Turkey Breakfast Sausage

1 pound ground turkey breast
1/3 cup unsweetened apple juice
1/4 teaspoon ham-flavored bouillon
4 tablespoons uncooked oatmeal
3/4 teaspoon crushed fennel seeds
1/4 teaspoon cracked pepper
1/8 teaspoon lite salt
cooking spray

Combine apple juice and bouillon in a large saucepan over low heat stir until granules are well dissolved. Add ground turkey, oatmeal and spices and mix well. Form into patties of equal size. Preheat a Teflon pan with cooking spray over medium heat. Place patties in Teflon pan and cook about 15 to 20 minutes or until browned. Turn each patty frequently and be sure to brown each side until cooked thoroughly. Makes 6 to 8 sausage patties.

Calories: 95 / Cholesterol: 70 milligrams / Protein: 13 grams / Fat: 0.5 gram / Fat: 5%

Sausage and Cheese Burrito

1 turkey sausage patty (see recipe above)
1 ounce shredded fat-free cheese
2 corn tortillas
Optional picante sauce

Place the turkey sausage patty between a folded moist paper towel and place in the microwave for 1 to 2 minutes or until heated. Crumble sausage into corn tortilla and place shredded cheese over sausage and top with picante sauce. Wrap and serve.

Calories: 240 / Cholesterol: 75 milligrams / Protein: 22 grams / Fat: 0.5 gram / Fat: 2%

Two Cheese Omelet

3 egg whites
1 ounce shredded fat-free cheddar cheese
1 ounce shredded fat-free mozzarella cheese

Spray a Teflon pan with butter flavored cooking spray, preheat on medium heat. Add egg whites and sprinkle cheese evenly over the center of the eggs. Cook until firm and fold. This is a good time to add additional things that your child likes. You can tailor the omelet to fit their individual taste. Add mushrooms, onions or whatever you know they will like. Serves 1.

Calories: 138 / Cholesterol: 20 milligrams / Protein: 20 grams / Fat: 0 / Fat: 0

Cheesy Spinach Potato

1/2 cup frozen spinach, cooked
1 cup mashed potato
1 ounce fat-free cheddar cheese, shredded
1 tablespoon fat-free Parmesan cheese

Preheat oven to 350 degrees. Thaw the spinach in the microwave and then puree. Take leftover mashed potatoes and stir in spinach, cheese and Parmesan. Place mixture in a baking dish that has been sprayed with butter flavored cooking spray. Bake in the oven for 15 to 18 minutes and serve.

Calories: 240 / Cholesterol: 0 / Protein: 4 grams / Fat: 1 gram / Fat: 4%

Lunch

Grilled Cheese Sandwich

2 slices fat-free cheese
2 slices lite whole wheat bread
Butter flavored cooking spray

Spray a Teflon pan with cooking spray and cook on medium heat. Place 1 slice of bread in pan and let that side brown. Place both slices of cheese on bread, top with other slice of bread and turn sandwich over. Let the bread brown, remove and serve.

Calories: 170 / Cholesterol: 0 / Protein: 15 grams / Fat: 0 / Fat: 0

Chicken Salad Sandwich

2 chicken breasts (cooked)
1/2 cup mustard
1/4 cup diced celery
1/4 cup diced red onion
1/2 teaspoon dill seasoning
Dill relish

Place all ingredients in a food processor. Blend until mixed. Place 3 ounces between two slices of lite whole wheat bread. Top with lettuce and tomato. Serves 3.

Calories: 115 / Cholesterol: 37 milligrams / Protein: 13 grams / Fat: 3.5 grams / Fat: 27%

Meatloaf Sandwich

(see meatloaf recipe under dinner recipes)
Take three ounces of meatloaf. Place between two slices of lite whole wheat bread. Top with catsup and lettuce and serve.

Calories: 195 / Cholesterol: 55 milligrams / Protein: 15 grams / Fat: 1 gram / Fat: 5%

Egg Salad Sandwich

2 slices lite whole wheat bread
3 hard boiled egg whites
2 tablespoons mustard
1 tablespoon fat-free mayonnaise
Dash dill seasoning
1 to 2 tablespoons dill relish
1 leaf lettuce

Mix all ingredients in a bowl. Toast bread. Place egg salad between two slices of toast and add lettuce.

Calories: 163 / Cholesterol: 0 / Protein: 14 grams / Fat: 1 gram / Fat: 6%

Tuna Salad Sandwich

2 slices lite whole wheat bread
3 ounce can water-packed tuna
2 tablespoons fat-free mayonnaise
1 stalk diced celery
1/4 diced small red onion
2 tablespoons dill relish
1 leaf lettuce
1 slice tomato

Drain and rinse water packed tuna. In a bowl mix together tuna, mayonnaise, celery, onion, and dill. Place tuna salad between the bread and layer the lettuce and tomato on tuna. (Tastes best if bread is toasted.)

Calories: 215 / Cholesterol: 37 milligrams / Protein: 22 grams / Fat: 1 gram / Fat: 4%

Cheese Sandwich

1 to 2 slices fat-free cheese
2 slices lite whole wheat bread
leaf lettuce
mustard
1 piece fresh fruit

Place the fat-free cheese between whole wheat bread, layer mustard on bread and cover with lettuce leaf. Serve with a piece of fresh fruit.

Calories: 230 / Cholesterol: 0 / Protein: 12 grams / Fat: 0 / Fat: 0

Potato Egg White Salad

6 ounce potato (cooked)
2 hard-boiled egg whites
dash dill seasoning
2 tablespoons mustard
1 celery stalk, diced
Dash pepper
Dash paprika
1 piece fresh fruit

Dice potato and egg whites and place in mixing bowl. Add dill, mustard, celery, pepper and paprika. Stir together well. Place in a Tupperware container and serve with fresh fruit on side.

Calories: 212 / Cholesterol: 0 / Protein: 10 grams / Fat: 1 gram / Fat: 4%

Turkey Salad Sandwich

8 ounces cooked turkey breast
1/4 cup mustard
2 diced scallions
Dill seasoning
2 stalks celery
1/4 cup diced water chestnuts
2 medium pita breads
Shredded lettuce and diced tomato

Place turkey breast, mustard, scallions, dill, celery and water chestnuts in food processor. Mix until all ingredients are shredded. Place turkey salad in pita pocket and top with lettuce and tomato. Serves 3 or 4.

Calories: 170 / Cholesterol: 38 milligrams /Protein: 16 grams / Fat: 1.5 grams / Fat: 8%

Chicken Sandwich

2 slices lite whole wheat bread
1 small chicken breast sliced
2 tablespoons fat-free mayonnaise
2 leaves lettuce
1 slice tomato
1 slice onion

Spread mayonnaise heavily on one side of each slice of bread. Place sliced chicken breast on bread. Top with lettuce, tomato and onion and serve.

Calories: 210 / Cholesterol: 50 milligrams / Protein: 16 grams / Fat: 3 grams / Fat: 13%

Chili

1 pound ground turkey breast
1 can Hunt's Mexican Style Tomato Sauce
1 can kidney beans, rinsed and drained
1 tablespoon chili powder
1/2 teaspoon garlic powder
Dash red pepper
1/2 cup shredded fat-free cheese

Over medium heat, brown the turkey breast while constantly working the meat with a wooden spoon to assure that the meat cooks in small pieces. Add the chili and garlic powder and red pepper. Add kidney beans, cover, let simmer for 10 minutes. Serves 4 or 5.

Calories: 250 / Cholesterol: 60 milligrams / Protein: 24 grams / Fat: 3 grams / Fat: 11%

Tuna Melt

6 ounce can water packed-tuna, drained
2 to 3 tablespoons fat-free mayonnaise
2 tablespoons dill relish
1 slice onion, diced fine
Small amount diced water chestnuts
4 whole wheat English muffin halves
4 slices fat-free cheddar or mozzarella cheese

Preheat oven to 375 degrees. Mix together tuna, mayonnaise. relish, onion and water chestnuts in a large mixing bowl. Toast English muffins. Place English muffin halves on a plate, top with tuna mixture and place a slice of cheese over the tuna. Place in preheated oven until cheese melts and serve. Serves 4.

Calories: 160 / Cholesterol: 25 milligrams / Protein: 17 grams / Fat: 1.5 grams / Fat: 6%

Nutritious Nibbling Snacks

Mini Pizza

1 whole wheat English muffin
1/4 cup tomato sauce
2 tablespoons fat-free Parmesan cheese
2 tablespoons fat-free cheese

Slice English muffin in half and toast. Coat each half with tomato sauce, Parmesan cheese and fat-free cheese. Place muffin halves in oven under broil for 3 to 4 minutes or until cheese melts. Serve.

Calories: 220 / Cholesterol: 0 / Protein: 5 grams / Fat: 1 gram / Fat: 4%

Frozen Grapes

1 cup grapes

Place grapes in freezer overnight. This is a great summer treat!

Calories: 120 / Cholesterol: 0 / Protein: 0 / Fat: 0 / Fat: 0

Fruit Smoothie

3/4 cup skim milk
3/4 cup ice
1/2 cup frozen strawberries
1/2 frozen banana

In a blender place milk, ice, fruit. Blend on high until smooth. Serve.

Calories: 190 / Cholesterol: 0 / Protein: 10 grams / Fat: 0 / Fat: 0

Banana Smoothie

3/4 cup skim milk
1/2 cup ice
2 frozen bananas
Dash cinnamon
1 package Equal

Place milk, ice, fruit and equal in a blender and blend on high until smooth. Pour into a large glass and sprinkle cinnamon on top and serve.

Calories: 260 / Cholesterol: 3 milligrams / Protein: 7 grams / Fat: 2 grams / Fat: 7%

Chocolate Milkshake

3/4 cup skim milk
3/4 cup ice
2 heaping tablespoons NutraSweet chocolate pudding mix

In a blender, mix together milk, ice and chocolate pudding mix until smooth and serve.

Calories: 125 / Cholesterol: 3 milligrams / Protein: 6 grams / Fat: 0 / Fat: 0

Cheese and Crackers

2 slices fat-free cheese
8 fat-free SnackWell crackers
6 ounces skim milk

Cut cheese slices in half. Fold cheese slices in half so that each slice of cheese is now twice as thick. Place fat-free cheese between crackers to make little finger-size sandwiches. Serve with a small glass of skim milk.

Calories: 215 / Cholesterol: 7 grams / Protein: 12 grams / Fat: 0 / Fat: 0

Cannonball Cantaloupe Balls

1/2 ripe cantaloupe
2 tablespoons Cool Whip Lite

With a melon ball scooper, scoop out cantaloupe and place in a small bowl. Be sure to stack the balls in a cannonball pyramid formation. Place Cool Whip over cannonballs and serve.

Calories: 140 / Cholesterol: 0 / Protein: 0 / Fat: 0 / Fat: 0

Yogurt, Oats and Raisins

1 lite yogurt, any flavor
1/4 cup uncooked oatmeal
2 tablespoons raisins

Mix all ingredients together in a Tupperware bowl. Place bowl in refrigerator for 30 minutes or longer. The oats will absorb the moisture from the yogurt to create a delightful flavor.

Calories: 195 / Cholesterol: 4 milligrams / Protein: 9 grams / Fat: 0 / Fat: 0

Nutty Yogurt

1 lite yogurt, any flavor
1/4 cup Grape Nuts cereal

Place the cereal in a bowl, and pour yogurt over cereal. Stir until yogurt and cereal are mixed. Serves 1.

Calories: 220 / Cholesterol: 12 milligrams / Protein: 14 grams / Fat: 0 / Fat: 0

Lemon Yogurt Sauce for Fruit

1 cup plain nonfat yogurt
1 tablespoon sugar or 1 package Equal
1 tablespoon lemon juice

In a small bowl, mix together all of the ingredients until well blended. Serve over a bed of any type of diced fruit. You can place this over strawberries, bananas, or melons, or put it on top of a medley of fruits.

Calories: 135 / Cholesterol: 0 / Protein: 11 grams / Fat: 0 / Fat: 0

Dinner

Chicken Fingers

1 pound boneless, skinless chicken breast
3/4 cup Kraft oil-free Italian dressing
1 cup corn flakes (crumbs)
Salt and pepper to taste
Dash Molly McButter

Slice chicken breast into strips and marinate in salad dressing for 1 to 2 hours (keep refrigerated). Remove chicken from marinade and roll breast in the corn flake crumbs. Place chicken strips on a nonstick cookie sheet. Bake at 400 degrees for approximately 35 minutes or until chicken is browned. Sprinkle with salt, pepper and Molly McButter to taste. Serves 4.

Calories: 212 / Cholesterol: 55 milligrams / Protein: 24 grams / Fat: 4 grams / Fat: 17%

Hawaiian Chicken

1 pound boneless, skinless chicken breast
1/4 teaspoon teriyaki sauce
1/4 teaspoon soy sauce
2 tablespoons lemon juice
1 fresh pineapple, diced (canned pineapple in own juices optional)
2 cups cooked rice

Mix together teriyaki sauce, soy sauce and lemon juice. Place chicken in marinade and let marinate in the refrigerator for 1 to 2 hours. Grill chicken breast. Place chicken breast over bed of rice and top with diced pineapple. Serves 4.

Calories: 270 / Cholesterol: 55 milligrams /Protein: 24 grams / Fat: 4 grams / Fat: 13%

Mango Shrimp

1 pound extra large shrimp
3 fresh mangos
3/4 cup orange juice
Dash nutmeg

Dice mango into small pieces and place in a large bowl. Add orange juice and nutmeg and stir well. Peel shrimp and grill dry. Place shrimp on plate and cover with mango mixture. Serves four or five.

Calories: 215 / Cholesterol: 130 milligrams / Protein: 17 grams / Fat: 2 grams / Fat: 8%

Turkey Burgers

1 pound ground turkey breast
3 egg whites
1/4 bread crumbs
1/4 diced onion
1/2 package dried vegetable soup mix
Dash garlic powder, garlic salt and pepper

In a large mixing bowl, mix all ingredients until well blended. Form into patties and grill over medium heat until thoroughly cooked. Serve with regular low fat condiments that would normally be served with any burger. Great with yam chips! Serves 4.

Calories: 183 / Cholesterol: 60 milligrams / Protein: 20 grams / Fat: 1 gram / Fat: 5%

Spicy Chicken

1 pound boneless, skinless chicken breast
1 cup low fat buttermilk
1 tablespoon Tabasco sauce
1 tablespoon soy sauce

Mix together buttermilk, Tabasco, and soy sauce. Cut chicken breast into strips. Place chicken breast in marinade (either overnight or for a few hours).

Coating:
1 cup cornmeal
1/4 teaspoon garlic powder
1/4 teaspoon cumin
1/4 teaspoon paprika
2 tablespoons Parmesan cheese

Mix cornmeal and seasonings well. Roll chicken breast in cornmeal mix and place on a Teflon baking sheet. Bake for 20 minutes at 425 degrees or until golden brown. Makes 6 servings.

Calories: 168 / Cholesterol: 66 milligrams / Protein: 14 grams / Fat: 2.2 grams / Fat: 11%

Chicken Fajitas

1 pound boneless, skinless chicken breast
1 white onion (sliced)
1 bell pepper (sliced)
Diced tomatoes and cilantro
8 corn tortillas
Molly McButter

Grill chicken dry and slice into strips. Spray a Teflon pan with Pam vegetable spray and cook onions and bell peppers over medium heat until tender. Sprinkle with Molly McButter. Remove from heat and place chicken, vegetables and diced tomatoes on separate plates. Let your child pick and choose what foods he or she would like to roll into the corn tortillas. Serves 5.

Calories: 214 / Cholesterol: 65 milligrams / Protein: 20 grams / Fat: 2.6 grams / Fat: 11%

Chicken, Rice and Vegetable Soup

1 cup water
7 1/2 ounce can tomatoes (1)
1 cup sliced carrots
1/2 cup chopped onion
1/4 cup chopped green pepper
2 teaspoons instant chicken bouillon granules
1/2 teaspoon dried thyme
1/4 teaspoon ground sage
1/8 teaspoon pepper
1 cup chopped chicken breast meat, cooked
1 cup cooked rice

In a saucepan combine all ingredients except chicken and rice. Bring to a boil, cover and simmer for 15 minutes. Stir in chicken and rice. Simmer for 10 more minutes, then serve. Makes 3 or 4 servings.

Calories: 70 / Cholesterol: 48 milligrams / Protein: 7 grams / Fat: 1 gram / Fat: 2%

This recipe makes a great meal if you add cooked rice or noodles into the soup right before serving.

Meatloaf

1 pound ground turkey breast
1 cup chopped onions
4 egg whites
1/2 cup barbecue sauce
1/2 cup ketchup
2/3 cup uncooked oatmeal
1 package Knorr vegetable soup mix
1/4 teaspoon pepper
1/2 teaspoon garlic powder

Preheat oven to 350 degrees. In a large mixing bowl mix all ingredients except ketchup until thoroughly blended. Place in meatloaf pan that has been sprayed with butter flavored cooking spray. Bake for about 60 to 90 minutes or until center is cooked thoroughly. Cover top of meatloaf with ketchup. Serves 8.

Calories: 122 / Cholesterol: 51 milligrams / Protein: 15 grams / Fat: 1.1 grams / Fat: 8%

Cheesy Lasagna

1 pound ground turkey breast
1/2 cup chopped onions
1/2 cup chopped celery
1/4 teaspoon pepper
1/2 teaspoon oregano
1/4 teaspoon garlic powder
12 ounces lasagna noodles
6 ounces fat-free cottage cheese
8 ounces shredded fat-free mozzarella cheese
6 ounce can tomato sauce
1 package chopped spinach

Brown turkey over medium heat and mix in onions, celery, pepper, oregano, and garlic powder. Boil lasagna noodles. Beginning with a layer of tomato sauce, layer ingredients in the following order in a large lasagna pan: noodles, meat, spinach, cottage cheese, tomato sauce. Repeat layers ending with a layer of noodles topped with tomato sauce. Cover with aluminum foil. Bake at 350 degrees for one hour. Serves 6 to 8.

Calories: 260 / Cholesterol: 75 milligrams / Protein: 26 grams / Fat: 1 gram / Fat: 4%

Turkey Meatballs

1 pound ground turkey breast
2 egg whites
3/4 cup soft bread crumbs
1/2 cup skim milk
1/4 cup chopped onion
1/2 teaspoon salt
Dash pepper
1/2 teaspoon dried oregano
1 tablespoon parsley

In a large bowl, combine egg whites, bread crumbs, milk, onion, salt, oregano, pepper, and parsley. Add ground turkey and mix together well. Shape 1/4 cup of meat mixture evenly into a ball. Place in baking dish sprayed with Pam and bake at 375 degrees for 25 to 30 minutes. Serve over a bed of pasta with tomato sauce. Makes 6 servings.

Calories: 104 / Cholesterol: 70 milligrams / Protein: 36 grams / Fat: 1 gram / Fat: 9%

Low Fat Nachos

1/2 pound ground turkey breast
5 ounces baked, fat-free tortilla chips
6 ounces fat-free refried beans
4 ounces fat-free cheddar cheese (shredded)
2 teaspoons chili powder
1/2 teaspoon garlic powder
1/4 diced onion (optional)

Over medium heat, brown the ground turkey breast seasoned with the chili powder, garlic powder and onion. Continually stir the turkey with a wooden spoon until all the turkey breast is thoroughly cooked. Reduce the heat and stir in the beans. Place a table-spoon of mixture on each chip and sprinkle with cheese. The heat from the mixture will melt the cheese. Serves 5.

Calories: 228 / Cholesterol: 19 milligrams /Protein: 17 grams / Fat: 2 grams / Fat: 8%

Spaghetti and Meatballs

16 ounce package pasta
1 jar low fat spaghetti sauce
1 pound ground turkey breast
2 egg whites
4 slices whole wheat bread (soaked in water, with excess squeezed out)
1/2 cup finely chopped onions
1/2 cup finely chopped celery
1/2 teaspoon garlic powder
1 tablespoon parsley
1/2 tablespoon basil
1/2 teaspoon pepper

In a large mixing bowl thoroughly mix turkey breast, egg whites, bread, onions, celery and spices. Form into balls (2-inch diameter). Place balls on cookie sheet and broil for approximately 10 to 15 minutes, turning occasionally until they are completely browned. Add meatballs into low fat spaghetti sauce and simmer over low heat for 1 1/2 hours. Boil pasta, drain and place meatballs and sauce over pasta. Serves 8.

Calories: 315 / Cholesterol: 51 milligrams / Protein: 21 grams / Fat: 4.3 grams / Fat: 12%

Sloppy Joes

1 pound ground turkey breast
1/2 diced onion
1 can Hunt's Italian tomato paste
1 can kidney beans
2 tablespoons chili powder
Dash garlic powder
4 whole wheat buns

Brown turkey breast over medium heat. Add tomato sauce, kidney beans, onion, chili and garlic powder. Cover, let simmer for 10 minutes. Place between buns and serve. Serves 4.

Calories: 236 / Cholesterol: 47 milligrams / Protein: 30 grams / Fat: 4 grams / Fat: 15%

Chicken Enchiladas

1 pound ground chicken breast
1 small onion, sliced
4 ounces shredded fat-free cheese
Green bell peppers
6 corn tortillas

Brown ground chicken breast. Sauté onions and green bell peppers over medium heat in a Teflon pan that has been sprayed with butter flavored cooking spray. Place ground chicken, onions, bell peppers and cheese in corn tortillas, wrap and serve. Serves 4 or 5.

Calories: 229 / Cholesterol: 55 milligrams /Protein: 32 grams / Fat: 4 grams / Fat: 16%

Macaroni and Cheese

1 1/2 tablespoons cornstarch
3/4 cup evaporated skim milk
3 raw egg whites
6 ounces fat-free cheddar cheese (shredded)
1/2 cup nonfat cottage cheese
10 ounces macaroni, cooked and drained

Preheat oven to 375 degrees. Mix together cornstarch and milk. Add egg whites and stir. Add the rest of the ingredients and stir well. Spray a medium size glass baking dish with cooking spray. Pour mixture into baking dish and place in oven. Bake approximately 25 minutes. Serves 5.

Calories: 298 / Cholesterol: 11 milligrams /Protein: 13 grams / Fat: 2 grams / Fat: 6%

Pirate Black Beans

1 can black beans, rinsed and drained
1 tomato, diced
1/2 diced red onion
1 cup frozen corn, thawed
2 tablespoons diced fresh cilantro

In a large mixing bowl stir together all ingredients and serve. Serves 3.

Calories: 150 / Cholesterol: 0 / Protein: 12 grams / Fat: 0 / Fat: 0

Unfried Shrimp

1 pound shrimp, peeled
4 egg whites
1 cup flour
1 teaspoon salt
1/2 teaspoon onion salt
1 teaspoon pepper

In a large plastic bag mix flour, salt, onion salt and pepper. Roll shrimp in egg whites. Place each shrimp in the bag and shake until shrimp is coated with flour mixture. Preheat a Teflon pan with butter flavored cooking spray over medium heat. Place shrimp in pan and cook until shrimp curl. Serves 4.

Calories: 236 / Cholesterol: 173 milligrams / Protein: 23 grams / Fat: 2 grams / Fat: 8%

Turkey Tacos

1 pound ground turkey breast
8 ounce can whole tomatoes (drained)
1 teaspoon chili powder
1/2 teaspoon cumin
1/4 teaspoon cayenne
2 tablespoons minced garlic
1/2 chopped medium onion
1/4 cup chopped celery
Shredded lettuce and 3/4 cup shredded fat-free cheese
Diced fresh tomatoes
8 to 10 corn tortillas

Brown turkey over medium heat in a nonstick skillet. Add tomatoes, onions, celery and spices. Cover, reduce heat and let simmer for 10 minutes. Place turkey taco meat into corn tortillas and top with lettuce, cheese and diced tomatoes. Serves 5.

Calories: 212 / Cholesterol: 50 milligrams / Protein: 16 grams / Fat: 1 gram / Fat: 4%

Orange Chicken

1 pound skinless chicken breast
1 cup orange juice
1 teaspoon oregano
1 teaspoon parsley
Dash garlic powder
Dash pepper
Orange wedges

Marinate breast in orange juice, oregano, parsley, garlic, and pepper for 6 hours. Remove chicken. Place on nonstick broiler rack. Broil until chicken is brown, baste with marinade occasionally. Place orange wedges on breast. Serve over a bed of rice. Serves 4.

Calories: 182 / Cholesterol: 97 milligrams / Protein: 20 grams / Fat: 2.2 grams / Fat: 11%

Mashed Potatoes

2 large red potatoes
3/4 cup skim milk
1/4 teaspoon garlic powder
1/4 teaspoon pepper
1 tablespoon onion bits
2 tablespoons fat-free Parmesan cheese
1/2 teaspoon Molly McButter
Dash parsley

Cook potatoes in microwave until well done. Place potatoes and all ingredients except parsley in a food processor or bowl and blend until smooth. Sprinkle parsley on each serving of potatoes. Makes 2 servings.

Calories: 170 / Cholesterol: 4 milligrams / Protein: 3 grams / Fat: 1 gram / Fat: 6%

Potato Twice Baked

1 large potato
1 tablespoon chives
4 tablespoons low fat cottage cheese
1 teaspoon Molly McButter
1/4 cup shredded fat-free Alpine Lace cheese
1 teaspoon parsley
2 tablespoons fat-free Parmesan cheese

Bake potato in oven at 450 degrees until done or nuke it in the microwave. Slice potato in half and remove insides and put potato skins on cookie sheet. Place potato insides in bowl and mash with chives, cottage cheese, Molly McButter and Alpine Lace cheese. Replace mixture in potato skins. Top with parsley and Parmesan cheese and place under broiler for 5 minutes. Serves 2.

Calories: 195 / Cholesterol: 10 milligrams / Protein: 7 grams / Fat: 1.5 grams / Fat: 7%

Potato Salad

3 cups cubed cooked potatoes
1/2 cup mustard
1/4 cup diced onions
1/4 teaspoon garlic salt
1/4 cup diced celery
1/4 teaspoon paprika
1/2 teaspoon dill

Place all ingredients in a large mixing bowl. Stir together and mix all ingredients well. Refrigerate leftovers. Serves 3.

Calories: 120 / Cholesterol: 0 / Protein: 8 grams / Fat: 1 gram / Fat: 7%

Potato Chips

Follow the same instructions as Yam Chips except use a potato and regular salt.

Yam Chips

1 large raw yam with skin removed
2 teaspoons garlic salt
Butter flavored cooking spray

Preheat oven to 400 degrees. Slice yam into thin slices and spread out over a cookie sheet that has been sprayed with butter flavored cooking spray. Sprinkle yam chips with garlic salt and place tray in oven. After 20 minutes, turn over chips and spray once again with cooking spray and sprinkle with garlic salt. Cook until chips are brown.

Calories: 200 / Cholesterol: 0 / Protein: 2 grams / Fat: 0 / Fat: 0

Marshmallow Yams

4 medium yams
3/4 cup skim milk
Butter Buds (equal to 1 1/2 tablespoons.)
1 package Equal
1/4 teaspoon cinnamon
1/4 teaspoon nutmeg
3/4 cup marshmallows

Place yams in microwave and cook on high until done. Remove skins and place insides in a food processor or blender with the milk, Butter Buds, Equal, cinnamon and nutmeg. Mix until smooth. Stir in marshmallows. Serves 4.

Calories: 136 / Cholesterol: 0 / Protein: 4 grams / Fat:.3 grams / Fat: 2%

French Fried Yams

2 large yams
Dash garlic powder
Dash Molly McButter
Dash lite salt

Preheat oven to 375 degrees. Spray a cookie sheet that has been lined with aluminum foil with butter flavored cooking spray. Slice the yams into long pieces and spread out evenly over cookie sheet. Sprinkle with spices. Place in oven and turn fries over when they appear browned. Cook until evenly browned. Serves 2.

Calories: 178 / Cholesterol: 0 / Protein: 3 grams / Fat: 0.2 grams / Fat: 1%

Oven Baked French Fries

1 large potato
3 large egg whites
1/4 cup flour
1 tablespoon Mrs. Dash
1 teaspoon lite salt
2 teaspoons chili powder

Preheat oven to 425 degrees. Slice potato in 1/4-inch slices. Mix flour and seasonings together. Dip potato slices in egg whites and then roll them in flour mixture. Place potato slices on Teflon cookie sheet that has been sprayed with butter flavored cooking spray. Place in oven and bake until golden brown. Turn 1 or 2 times. Serves 2.

Calories: 114 / Cholesterol: 0 / Protein: 3 grams / Fat: 0.3 grams / Fat: 2%

Cherry Rice

2 cups chicken broth
1 cup rice
1/2 cup dried cherries

Place broth in saucepan and bring to a boil. Add uncooked rice, reduce heat and cover. Let simmer over low heat until rice absorbs broth. Remove from heat. Stir in cherries and serve. Serves 3.

Calories: 170 / Cholesterol: 0 / Protein: 2 grams / Fat: 2 grams / Fat: 10%

Corny Rice

1 cup uncooked rice
2 cups chicken broth
1 cup frozen corn

Bring chicken broth to a boil, add rice. Reduce heat, cover and let simmer until rice is tender. Toss in frozen corn, cover and let simmer for 5 more minutes. Stir well and serve. Serves 3.

Calories: 200 / Cholesterol: 0 / Protein: 2 grams / Fat: 2 grams / Fat: 9%

Oven Fried Zucchini

1 large zucchini
3 egg whites
3 tablespoons flour
1/4 cup bread crumbs
3 tablespoons fat-free Parmesan cheese

Preheat oven to 375 degrees. Mix together flour, bread crumbs and Parmesan cheese. Slice zucchini. Dip zucchini in egg white and roll it in the flour mixture until it is coated with batter. Place slices on a cookie sheet that has been sprayed with butter flavored cooking spray. Spread evenly. Place in oven for 20 minutes or until golden brown, turn and let cook until golden brown. Serves 2.

Calories: 95 / Cholesterol: 0 / Protein: 6 grams / Fat: 1 gram / Fat: 10%

Potato Bake

4 large baking potatoes, cooked, peeled and diced
4 ounces fat-free cream cheese
4 ounces fat-free cheddar cheese (shredded)
3/4 cup nonfat cottage cheese
1 tablespoon cornstarch
Dash pepper
Dash garlic powder
1 teaspoon salt
3/4 package Butter Buds
1/4 cup artificial bacon bits

Mash potatoes in a large bowl. Add remaining ingredients and mix well. Pour mixture into a casserole dish that has been sprayed with cooking spray. Bake for 25 minutes or until browned. Serves 4 to 6.

Calories: 315 / Cholesterol: 20 milligrams /Protein: 11 grams / Fat: 3 grams / Fat: 8%

Cheesy Zucchini

1 large zucchini, sliced
8 ounce can tomato sauce
4 ounces fat-free cheddar cheese (shredded)
4 tablespoons fat-free Parmesan cheese

Preheat oven to 375 degrees. In a mixing bowl, mix together zucchinis, tomato sauce and shredded cheese. Place in oven for 15 minutes. Top with Parmesan cheese and place under broiler until Parmesan cheese is lightly browned. Serves 2.

Calories: 145 / Cholesterol: 0 / Protein: 15 grams / Fat: 0 / Fat: 0

Desserts

Spicy Popcorn

1/4 cup uncooked popcorn
1 tablespoon fat-free Parmesan cheese
Butter flavored cooking spray
Dash lite salt
1 tablespoon chili powder

Air pop the popcorn. Place half of air-popped popcorn in a bowl and sprinkle with half the seasonings over popcorn. Lightly spray with cooking spray so that the seasoning sticks. Repeat the process with the other half of popcorn and spices.

Calories: 50 / Cholesterol: 0 / Protein: .8 grams/ Fat: .3grams / Fat:5%

Baked Apple

1 apple
1 teaspoon brown sugar
1/4 teaspoon Molly McButter
Dash cinnamon
1 tablespoon raisins (optional)
Dash Cool Whip Lite

Core apple. Sprinkle into core a mixture of sugar, Molly McButter, dash cinnamon, and raisins. Place in baking dish and bake uncovered for 30 minutes at 350 degrees. (Be sure to add a small amount of water in baking dish to prevent sticking.) Remove from oven, let cool and top with Cool Whip. Serves 1.

Calories: 100 / Cholesterol: 0 / Protein: 1 gram / Fat: 0 / Fat: 0

Cool Yogurt

1 carton lite yogurt (any flavor)
2 heaping tablespoons Cool Whip Lite
2 tablespoons crushed graham crackers
Sprinkle of chocolate

In a medium bowl, mix together yogurt and Cool Whip. Let sit in refrigerator for at least one hour or over night. Sprinkle with graham cracker crumbs and and chocolate and serve. Serves 1.

Calories: 180 / Cholesterol: 0 / Protein: 12 grams / Fat: 1 gram / Fat: 5%

Homemade Vanilla Frozen Yogurt

1 pint nonfat vanilla yogurt
2 1/2 tablespoons liquid fructose
1/4 teaspoon vanilla extract

Mix all ingredients together by whisking until well blended. Freeze in an ice cream maker according to manufacturer's directions. Serve immediately, or place in a sealed container in the freezer.
*Note: You can alter this recipe to make any flavor yogurt desired. Just add any flavor low sugar jam or preserves into mixture. Use about 2 to 3 tablespoons Serves 2.

Calories: 130 / Cholesterol: 0 / Protein: 6 grams / Fat: 0 / Fat: 0

Banana Chocolate Mousse

2 1/4 cups cold skim milk
1/2 package sugar free Jell-O instant chocolate pudding mix
1/2 package sugar free Jell-O instant banana pudding mix
1 1/2 cups Cool Whip Lite

Mix together milk and pudding mix. With a wire whisk or low speed mixer, beat until well blended. Fold in Cool Whip with a spoon until evenly mixed. Place mixture in wine glasses and place in the refrigerator for at least 30 minutes. Makes 8, 1/2-cup servings.

Calories: 76 / Cholesterol: 9 milligrams / Protein: 2 grams / Fat: 0 / Fat: 0

Chocolate Brownies

2/3 cup unbleached all-purpose flour
1/2 cup unsweetened cocoa
1/2 teaspoon baking powder
1/4 teaspoon salt
1/3 cup lite margarine
1 cup sugar
3 large egg whites
1 teaspoon vanilla extract

Preheat oven to 350 degrees. Spray an 8-inch square pan with nonstick cooking spray. Combine the flour, cocoa powder, baking powder and salt. Set aside. Cream margarine and sugar. Beat in egg whites and vanilla. Gradually add in the flour mixture, stirring until well blended. Spread the batter in the pan, and bake for about 30 minutes or until a toothpick inserted in the center comes out clean. Let brownies cool. Makes 16 brownies.

Calories: 95 / Cholesterol: 1 milligram / Protein: 2 grams / Fat: 2 grams / Fat: 18%

Apple, Cherry, Raisin Brownies

1 1/2 cups flour
2 teaspoons baking powder
1/3 cup lite margarine
1 cup brown sugar
1/2 cup sugar
3 egg whites
1 teaspoon vanilla extract
1 cup peeled, cored and chopped red apple
1/3 cup applesauce
1/4 cup dried cherries
3 tablespoons raisins

Preheat oven to 350 degrees. Spray an 8-inch square pan with nonstick cooking spray. In a large bowl, combine flour and baking soda. Set aside. Cream margarine with a mixer. Gradually add brown and white sugar. Beat in the egg. Add in the flour mixture. Stir in the vanilla, apples, applesauce, cherries and raisins. Evenly pour the mixture into the pan, and bake for about 35 minutes, or until a toothpick inserted in the center comes out clean. Makes 15 brownies.

Calories: 100 / Cholesterol: 0 / Protein: 2 grams / Fat: 1.2 grams / Fat: 11%

Root Beer Float

3/4 cup lite, low fat vanilla ice cream
1 can diet root beer
Large mug

Place ice cream in large mug. Slowly pour root beer over ice cream and serve.

Calories: 90 / Cholesterol: 20 milligrams / Protein: 6 grams / Fat: 2 grams / Fat: 20%

Chocolate Marshmallow Brownies

3/4 cup cake flour
1/2 cup cocoa
2 teaspoons baking soda
1/4 cup lite margarine, melted
2 cups sugar
4 egg whites
3 tablespoons vanilla extract
1 cup mini-marshmallows

Preheat oven to 325 degrees. Spray an 8-inch pan with nonstick cooking spray. Sift together flour, cocoa and baking powder. Set aside. With a mixer, cream the margarine and sugar until blended. Add egg whites and beat well. Stir in vanilla. Gradually stir in flour mixture until thoroughly combined. Fold in marshmallows. Evenly spread the mixture into the baking pan and bake for about 30 minutes or until a toothpick inserted at the edge comes out clean. The center is supposed to be slightly soft. Makes 15 brownies.

Calories: 100 / Cholesterol: 0 / Protein: 2 grams / Fat: 1.2 grams / Fat: 10%

Cocoa Chewies
3 egg whites
3/4 cup sugar
2 teaspoons water
1 teaspoon vanilla
3 tablespoons cocoa powder
Butter flavored cooking spray

Preheat oven to 250 degrees. Whip egg whites until stiff (but not dry). Slowly add 1/2 cup of sugar while you continue to whip the egg whites. In a separate bowl, mix together water and vanilla. Add water and vanilla mixture slowly to egg whites. Slowly add the rest of the sugar while you continue to whip egg whites. Stop whipping and fold in cocoa powder by hand. Be gentle and fold in carefully. Drop mixture by heaping tablespoon full onto a cookie sheet that has been sprayed with butter flavored cooking spray. Be sure to leave space between each spoonful. Bake for 35 to 40 minutes.

Calories: 52 / Cholesterol: 0 / Protein: 1 gram / Fat: 0 / Fat: 0

Chocolate Chip Marshmallow Cookies

4 egg whites
1 cup packed brown sugar
1 1/3 cup all purpose flour
1 cup mini-marshmallows
1/4 teaspoon baking powder
1/4 teaspoon salt
2/3 cup semisweet chocolate chips

Preheat oven to 375 degrees. Spray cookie sheet with nonstick cooking spray. In a large bowl, mix together egg whites and sugar until well blended. In a separate bowl, mix together the flour, baking powder and salt. Add egg mixture and marshmallow and stir together. Add in chocolate chips. Place the dough by rounded teaspoons about 1 1/2 inches apart on cookie sheet. Bake 7 minutes or until cookies begin to brown around the edges. Makes 5 to 6 dozen.

Calories: 30 / Cholesterol: 6 milligrams / Protein: 0.4 grams / Fat: 0.5 grams / Fat: 15%

Fat Free Rice Krispy Treats

2 tablespoons skim milk
4 cups mini-marshmallows
1 half ounce packet Butter Buds
6 cups Rice Krispies
1 cup raisins

Spray a 13 x 9 inch pan with butter flavored cooking spray. Place the skim milk and marshmallows in a saucepan and cook over low heat and allow everything to melt. Stir often. When marshmallows are melted, stir in Butter Buds. When well mixed, remove from heat and stir in Rice Krispies and raisins. Press the mixture into the pan and spread evenly. Allow to cool and serve.

Calories: 110 / Cholesterol: 0 / Protein: 1.5 grams / Fat: 0 / Fat: 0

Oatmeal Raisin Cookies

2 1/2 cups whole wheat flour
1 cup raw oatmeal
1 teaspoon baking soda
1 teaspoon ground cinnamon
1/2 teaspoon ground ginger
1/4 teaspoon nutmeg
1/4 teaspoon salt
1/2 cup lite margarine
1/2 cup brown sugar
1/2 cup molasses
2 large egg whites
1/2 cup chopped raisins

In a large bowl, mix flour, oatmeal, baking soda, cinnamon, ginger, nutmeg and salt. In a separate bowl, mix together margarine and sugar until smooth. Gradually add flour mixture. Stir in chopped raisins. Gather the dough and form into one large ball. Wrap ball of dough in plastic wrap and refrigerate for about one hour. Preheat oven to 375 degrees. Spray cookie sheets with nonstick cooking spray. Remove dough from refrigerator. Pinch off evenly sized amounts of dough and roll into balls. Place on cookie sheet and flatten each ball. Bake for about 15 minutes or until the tops are slightly puffed and crack. Makes 4 to 5 dozen.

Calories: 60 / Cholesterol: 0 / Protein: 1 gram / Fat: 0.8 gram / Fat: 12%

Lemon Icebox Cookies

2 cups unbleached flour
1/4 cup wheat germ
1/4 teaspoon salt
1/4 teaspoon baking soda
1/2 cup lite margarine
1 cup sugar
2 large egg whites
3 tablespoons freshly squeezed lemon juice
1 teaspoon lemon zest

In a large bowl, mix flour, wheat germ, salt and baking soda. In a separate bowl, using an electric mixer on high speed, cream butter and sugar. Add egg whites, lemon juice and zest and beat until blended. Gradually stir in the flour mixture. Divide the dough into two equal portions and form each into a log two inches in diameter. Wrap the logs in plastic wrap and refrigerate for at least 3 hours. Preheat the oven to 400 degrees. Cut slices (about 1/8 inch thick) off the logs and place them on cookie sheets that have been sprayed with nonstick cooking spray. Bake 12 to 14 minutes, or until lightly browned on edges. Makes about 6 dozen.

Calories: 31 / Cholesterol: 0 / Protein: 0.6 gram / Fat: 0.8 gram / Fat: 22%

Blueberry Muffins

2 cups flour
4 teaspoons baking soda
3/4 cup sugar
1 teaspoon salt
1 cup canned blueberries
4 egg whites
1/2 cup melted lite margarine
1 cup skim milk

Preheat oven to 400 degrees. Sift together flour, baking powder, sugar and salt. Add berries and stir until well coated. In a separate bowl, beat egg whites, milk and melted margarine and once mixed, add to dry mixture. Stir until blended. Fill muffin tins 3/4 full. Bake for 20 minutes or until brown.

Calories: 173 / Cholesterol: 5 milligrams / Protein: 2 grams / Fat: 4 grams / Fat: 21%

Chocolate Angel Food Cake

1 1/2 cups sifted flour
1 3/4 cup sugar
14 egg whites
1 teaspoon cream of tartar
2 teaspoons vanilla extract
1/2 teaspoon almond extract
1 1/2 teaspoons lemon juice
1 package chocolate Nutra-Sweetened pudding

Preheat oven to 300 degrees. Sift flour into mixing bowl. Sift sugar into a separate bowl. Set aside. Beat egg whites until foamy. Add cream of tartar and continue to mix until the egg whites form soft peaks. Gently fold in sugar. Gently fold in flour a little at a time. Mix together vanilla, almond and lemon juice in a separate bowl. Slowly add mixture into the egg white mixture. Pour into a 10-inch tube pan and bake about 1 hour or until light brown. The top should spring back when touched. Let cool upside down in the pan. When ready to serve, run a knife between the pan and cake and gently remove.

Topping: Make the pudding according to package directions using skim milk. Drizzle the pudding mixture over the top of the cake before serving. Makes 12 slices.

Calories: 225 / Cholesterol: 0 / Protein: 5 grams / Fat 0 / Fat 0

Raisin Carrot Cookies

2 1/2 cups all purpose flour
1 1/2 teaspoons ground ginger
1/2 teaspoon baking soda
1/2 teaspoon salt
1/4 teaspoon nutmeg
1/2 cup lite margarine
3/4 cup brown sugar
2 large egg whites
1 teaspoon vanilla extract
1 cup grated carrots
1/2 cup golden raisins

Preheat oven to 375 degrees. Spray cookie sheets with nonstick cooking spray. In a large bowl, stir together flour, ginger, baking soda, salt and nutmeg. In separate bowl, cream margarine and sugar. Beat in egg whites and vanilla. Gradually add in the flour mixture until blended. Stir in raisins and carrots. Drop dough by tablespoonfuls onto cookie sheets. Bake 12 to 14 minutes or until golden brown. Makes about 4 dozen.

Calories: 50 / Cholesterol: 0 / Protein: 0.8 grams / Fat: 1 gram / Fat: 19%

Banana Bread

2 1/4 cups sifted, unbleached flour
1 teaspoon baking powder
1/8 teaspoon salt
1/2 cup lite margarine
1 teaspoon baking soda
1 cup sugar
3 ripe bananas
4 egg whites
3/4 cup skim milk mixed with 3 teaspoons lemon juice

Preheat oven to 350 degrees. Sift together all dry ingredients and set aside. Blend margarine, milk and sugar until creamy. Add egg whites and mashed bananas into milk mixture and mix together thoroughly. Add the dry ingredients and stir briefly. Pour ingredients into floured loaf pans that have been sprayed with cooking spray. Bake 45 to 50 minutes or until toothpick comes out clean.

Calories: 150 / Cholesterol: 0 / Protein: 4 grams / Fat: 4 grams / Fat: 24%

Ambrosia

1 orange
1/2 cantaloupe
1 cup seedless grapes
1 banana
1/4 cup shredded coconut
2/3 cup orange juice

Peel the orange, cantaloupe and banana. Dice the fruit and add the grapes. Sprinkle coconut over the top. Pour the juice over the ambrosia and chill before serving. Serves 4.

Calories: 261 / Cholesterol: 11 grams / Protein: 1 gram / Fat: 9 grams / Fat: 31%

Gingerbread

2 1/2 cup unbleached flour
2 teaspoons baking soda
1 teaspoon cinnamon
1 teaspoon ground ginger
1 teaspoon mixed spice
1 cup skim milk
1/2 cup light molasses
1/2 cup sugar
1/2 cup lite margarine

Preheat oven to 350 degrees. Sift together all the dry ingredients. In a separate saucepan, warm the milk, sugar, molasses and margarine while stirring frequently. Do not let boil. Cool, add dry ingredients and stir until blended. Be careful not to overstir. Pour into a floured loaf pan that has been sprayed with cooking spray. Bake for 45 minutes or until toothpick comes out clean.

Calories: 182 / Cholesterol: 0 / Protein: 2 grams / Fat: 4 grams / Fat: 20%

Apple Surprise

3/4 cup unsweetened applesauce
1/4 cup mini-marshmallows
Dash cinnamon

Place applesauce in a bowl, sprinkle with cinnamon. Top with marshmallows and serve. Serves 2.

Calories: 140 / Cholesterol: 0 / Protein: 1 gram / Fat: 0 / Fat: 0

Popsicles

Purchase a popsicle mold and popsicle sticks. Pour your child's favorite juice in mold and freeze.

Beverages

Other than water, these beverages are great substitutes for regular sodas and too much juice.

- Try mixing 1/2 cup of your child's favorite juice with 1 cup of club soda. By using grape juice and club soda you will be creating grape soda. This works well with apple juice as well.

- If your child likes regular sodas, try finding a diet soda to substitute. Keep in mind that tastes change over time. In the beginning, you may have to mix half regular soda with diet until you can make the full switch.

- Try Nutra-Sweetened Kool-Aid or Crystal Light.

- Most health food stores sell decaffeinated herbal tea blends with strong fruit flavors. These can be made into iced tea. They make mango, blueberry, apricot and a host of other tea blends that kids find really refreshing.

- For a great fizz, try taking Crystal Light powder, place about one teaspoon in a tall glass and cover with club soda and ice.

Chocolate Milk

1 cup skim milk
1 1/2 teaspoons cocoa powder
2 packets Equal

Place skim milk in a blender with cocoa powder and Equal. Blend on high for 25 seconds and serve.

Calories: 100 / Cholesterol: 15 milligrams /Protein: 10 grams / Fat: 0 / Fat: 0

Hot Cocoa

1 cup skim milk
1 tablespoon honey
1 teaspoons cocoa powder
Drop of vanilla
2 tablespoons mini-marshmallows

Place cocoa, honey and 2 tablespoons milk in a cup and stir until mixed smoothly. Slowly add remaining skim milk. Place in microwave on high for 2 minutes. Add vanilla, stir and top with marshmallows.

Calories: 179 / Cholesterol: 0 / Protein: 10 grams / Fat: 0 / Fat: 0

Strawberry Blitz

10 ounces diet strawberry soda
1/2 cup skim milk
3/4 cup frozen strawberries
2 tablespoons Cool Whip Lite

Place soda, milk and strawberries in a blender and mix on medium until smooth. Pour into a tall mug and top with Cool Whip.

Calories: 197 / Cholesterol: 0 / Protein: 5 grams / Fat: 0 / Fat: 0

Orange Fizz

10 ounces diet orange soda
1 fresh orange, peeled
1/2 cup skim milk
2 tablespoons Cool Whip Lite

In a blender, mix soda, milk and orange until smooth. Pour into a tall mug and top with Cool Whip.

Calories: 115 / Cholesterol: 10 milligrams / Protein: 4 grams / Fat: 0 / Fat: 0

Strawberry Smoothie

1 cup frozen strawberries
1 carton plain nonfat yogurt
1/2 cup ice
1/2 cup skim milk
2 packets Equal

Place all ingredients in a blender and mix until smooth.

Calories: 255 / Cholesterol: 5 milligrams / Protein: 17 grams / Fat: 0 / Fat: 0

Banana Smoothie

2 frozen bananas
1 cup skim milk
2 packets Equal
Dash cinnamon

Place all ingredients except cinnamon in a blender and mix until smooth. Pour into a tall mug and top with cinnamon.

Calories: 330 / Cholesterol: 10 milligrams / Protein: 10 grams / Fat: 0 / Fat: 0

Banana Health Shake

1 carton lite banana yogurt
1/2 cup skim milk
1/2 cup ice
1/2 fresh banana

Mix all ingredients in a blender and mix until smooth. Pour into a tall mug and serve.

Calories: 195 / Cholesterol: 10 milligrams / Protein: 15 grams / Fat: 0 / Fat: 0

Orange Sherbet Punch

1 pint orange sherbet
2 cups orange juice
4 cups club soda
1 1/2 cups diced fresh strawberries

Mix together fruit juice and club soda in a punch bowl. Place strawberries and sherbet in bowl and stir in a circle five times or just until sherbet begins to melt.

Calories: 220 / Cholesterol: 0 / Protein: 0 / Fat: 0 / Fat: 0

Apple Fizz

1 cup apple juice
1 cup club soda
1/2 cup low sugar applesauce
1/2 cup ice

Place apple juice, ice and applesauce in a blender and mix until smooth. Pour in club soda and serve.

Calories: 210 / Cholesterol: 0 / Protein: 0 / Fat: 0 / Fat: 0

Kitchen Measurement Conversion Tables

The following conversion tables are intended to help you develop better cooking skills. They should allow you to convert many of your own recipes into lower fat meals. If your recipe uses a measurement that differs from the ones I use in this cookbook, simply use the conversion table to convert the recipe.

For example, if your old, high fat recipe called for 4 tablespoons of regular butter, you might substitute 4 tablespoons of lite margarine instead. On the other hand let's say that you found a really neat low fat recipe in this book that you wanted to try. However, when you searched your kitchen for your 1/3-cup measuring cup, you discovered that your child lost it while playing in the sandbox. Using the conversion table, you would discover that 1/3 of a cup equals 5 1/3 tablespoons.

You may also use the conversion tables to help you read labels. Many labels today list grams rather than teaspoons, cups, or quarts. For example, a cookie box states that one serving is 56 grams. Using the conversion table, you can convert grams into ounces. Since 1 ounce is equal to 28 grams, the serving size is equal to 2 ounces (56 divided by 28 equals 2 ounces).

Once again, another use of the conversion tables is to determine the number of teaspoons of sugar in foods. Since 4 grams equal 1 teaspoon, a food with 39 grams of sugar contains 9 3/4 teaspoons of sugar (39 divided by 4 equals 9.75 teaspoons).

To determine the percentage of fat in foods, locate the Calories From Fat on the Nutrition Facts Panel on the label and divide that number by the total calories listed on the panel. Drop the decimal point before the number and that is the percentage of fat. For example, 9 fat calories divided by 100 calories equals 0.09. Now, drop the decimal point. The food is 9 percent fat!

Using these tables is an easy way to convert your favorite recipes and to determine the sugar and fat content of the foods you buy.

Teaspoon	=	Tablespoon	=	Cup	=	Fluid Ounce
1	=	1/3			=	1/6
3	=	1			=	1/2
		2	=	1/8	=	1
		4	=	1/4	=	2
		5 1/3	=	1/3	=	2 2/3
		8	=	1/2	=	4
		10 2/3	=	2/3	=	5 1/3
		12	=	3/4	=	6
		14	=	7/8	=	7
		16	=	1	=	8

1 teaspoon = 4 grams

1 pint = 2 cup

1 quart = 2 pints

1 gallon = 4 quarts

1 gram = 0.035 ounce

1 ounce = 28 grams

1 pound = 16 ounces

1 kilogram = 2.21 pounds

Substitution List for Modifying Recipes

By using low fat substitutions a person can turn a high fat recipe into a low fat one without sacrificing taste, creating a Better Bad Choice. For example, let's suppose that your recipe calls for a cup of regular mayonnaise, which would add 1600 calories and 176 grams of fat to the recipe. Replace it with a cup of fat-free mayonnaise and you will reduce the calories to 320 and reduce the fat to 0. This simple substitution removes 1280 calories and 176 grams of fat from the recipe. Similarly, substituting skim milk for whole milk will reduce calories and fat significantly.

If you are not ready to try fat-free products, trying lite products can still make a big difference. For example, if your recipe calls for 4 tablespoons of butter, which have 400 calories and 45 grams of fat, and you use lite margarine instead, which has only 200 calories and 22 grams of fat, you have made a Better Bad Choice without changing the taste.

The following list contains suggested substitutions that you can make to your favorite recipes (ones you and your family have been eating for years). Naturally, you can't make all the substitutions all the time. However, if you learn these simple techniques, you will be surprised to find out how many calories and how much fat you can cut out of everyday recipes.

One word of caution: When you try these substitutions, don't tell anyone in your family; otherwise they will likely moan and complain because they think less fat means less flavor. The problem is that people have preconceived notions about low fat meals. Although they may have never tasted real low fat cooking, they may decide to hate it before ever really giving it a try. By not telling them until after they have eaten the meal, you will be more likely to hear their honest opinion about how the meal tastes. Try keeping it a secret for about a week. You'll notice no one complains or notices a change in flavor. It's interesting what people will do and say if they know ahead of time that you're going to be changing their favorite foods.

Here's another example of preconceived notions and their effect on people. A local radio station was moving into a new building. When the building's other tenants found out that the station was going into an office on the floor above them, they complained to the building owners. They were concerned that a radio station would make too much noise and be distracting. The station spent thousands of dollars on additional sound proofing to alleviate any potential problems. In spite of these efforts the tenants continued to complain to the landlord and sent out petitions attempting to block the station from moving in. Before the first sound check, the station sent memos to all the tenants letting them know the date and the time it would take place. On the date that the sound check was scheduled, the station had an electrical problem and could not conduct the sound test. Nevertheless, the next day the landlord received fifty-two complaints of excessive noise from a sound check that never took place!

By taking your family's favorite recipes and using lower fat ingredients, you will be creating Better Bad Choices and contributing to your family's overall health.

1.   If a recipe calls for a cream sauce, substitute tomato sauce.

2.   Rather than using cream soup in a recipe, replace it with nonfat dry milk.

3.   Substitute skim milk for whole milk or evaporated milk.

4.   Instead of using ice cream in a dessert, use nonfat frozen yogurt.

5.   When a recipe calls for regular butter or margarine, use diet margarine instead.

6.   Anytime a recipe calls for regular mayonnaise try an equal amount of a fat-free variety.

7.   If you use high fat dairy creamer in your coffee, switch to nonfat dry milk.

8.   When a recipe calls for nuts, replace them with a low fat granola.

9.   If a recipe calls for oils when baking, like in cakes or muffins, substitute unsweetened applesauce.

10.   Instead of using oils when frying, try using cooking spray.

11.   Rather than sautéing in oil, try low fat chicken broth.

12.   If a recipe calls for peanut butter, try apple butter instead.

13.   Replace regular salad dressings with one of the many fat-free versions.

14.   Use fat-free sour cream or nonfat plain yogurt rather than regular sour cream.

15.   If you want to use whipped cream, try fat free Cool Whip. It has a lot less fat.

16.   Whenever a recipe calls for a whole egg, replace it with 2 egg whites. Your family will never know the difference.

17.   Regular cream cheese can be replaced with a lite or fat-free version.

18.   When a recipe calls for avocado, use pureed asparagus.

19.   If your recipe needs bacon, try using Canadian bacon or Bacon Bits.

20.   Beef recipes can be conveniently altered using chicken or turkey breast without the skin.

21.   Rather than cooking rice with butter, try cooking it with chicken broth instead of water. Then add Molly McButter, after it's cooked.

22.   If a recipe calls for regular cheese, try using fat-free cheese. The key is to place the cheese in the dish immediately after removing the dish from the stove or oven.

23.   Replace potato chips and regular tortilla chips with baked chips.

24.   One ounce of baking chocolate can be replaced with 3 to 4 tablespoons of cocoa plus 1 teaspoon canola oil.

25.   If you need a chocolate sauce try mixing cocoa and apple juice.

26.   Defat meat broths and meat juices by chilling them in the refrigerator until the fat congeals on the top. Then remove the layer of fat.

27.   Substitute ground turkey breast for ground beef when making burgers, chili, meatloaf, tacos or spaghetti.

28.   To make fat-free gravies and sauces, brown flour in an iron skillet until it has a caramel color. Turn off the heat, and continue stirring until the flour cools. Mix the browned flour with meat juices or broths that you have defatted. Heat to a boil while stirring. Presto, you have a fat-free gravy.

29.   Grill rather than sauté, and sauté rather than deep-fry. Better yet, broil, poach or bake the meat on a rack so the meat isn't sitting in its own fatty juices.

30.   Air-pop popcorn as opposed to cooking it in oil. Rather than using butter, try spraying the popcorn with butter flavored cooking spray so that your toppings of cajun seasoning or fat-free Parmesan cheese will stick to the popcorn.

31.   Instead of using higher fat fish, use a lower fat one. Avoid salmon, catfish, and swordfish. Substitute flounder, red snapper, tuna steaks, shrimp, lobster and scallops.

Appendix I

Better Bad Choices for Fast Foods

It was no great surprise when McDonald's replaced its lower fat McLean sandwiches with the super-high-fat Arch Deluxe. Similarly, Taco Bell reduced the selection of Border Lights, which feature half the fat of their regular products and fewer calories, from eight items to three. And after an initial fanfare, Kentucky Fried Chicken discontinued its Rotisserie Gold chicken.

I wasn't surprised, because people who actively manage their weight and health don't eat in fast food restaurants. The failure to sell these lower fat items doesn't mean that the public doesn't want them. It simply indicates that offering healthy food isn't enough to draw truly health-minded people into the taco, chicken, and burger establishments.

Fast food is junk food, but if your child is already hooked, your goal should be to manage the junk food, not avoid it. Don't make a habit of eating fast food every week. Save it for special occasions such as birthdays or travel stops. Most fast food is very high in fat and the temptation to order fries and a regular soda can be pretty hard to resist, especially when your child is excited and hungry. Even though I oppose serving fast food to children, I also understand that circumstances may occasionally be beyond your control. Sometimes it's either fast food or no food. In this case, your only hope to help your son lose weight depends on your ability to help him make Better Bad Choices.

When you prepare food at home, focus on the percentage of fat and try to keep most meals below 20 percent. When you go out to eat, employ the Better Bad Choices philosophy and do the best you can. Eating out requires some compromises. The Better Bad Choices philosophy emphasizes flexibility and "doing better." Using Better Bad

Choices allows you and your kids to go out to eat occasionally without blowing the whole program.

Set a good example for your kids and remember to be consistent. Let your son have a burger, but leave off the mayonnaise, cheese, and bacon. Present a couple of Better Bad Choices to help him learn how to choose wisely. For example, offer a burger or a grilled chicken sandwich. If he chooses the burger, order a small one without the high fat condiments. Another way to make a Better Bad Choice would be to order smaller versions of the foods he normally eats. Opting for a small order of fries instead of a large will reduce overall fat and calories. Occasionally allow your child to splurge, but don't allow these splurges to undermine your overall plan. Prepare great, low fat food for the following few days to offset the fast-food meal.

Planning ahead is the key to success. The following list of fast foods shows you at a glance the amount of fat and calories in the foods offered by the major fast food chains. Preview the menu at the restaurant where you will be dining, and decide ahead of time which choices are better. If your children are old enough, let them look over the list. Encourage them to make selections that are lower in fat and calories. By letting your children have control over their Better Bad Choices, you will be teaching them responsibility and the decision making process. Although fast food contains an astronomical amount of calories, cholesterol, fat, and sodium, your kids will learn to make better choices and come out feeling good about their decisions. Success comes when your daughter says, "I made a much better choice today than I used to," instead of saying, "I'm so rotten for eating fast food."

Be wary of fast-food salads. They may not be a safe bet, because most kids (and adults) pile on the cheese and regular salad dressing. Many dressings contain more than a hundred calories per tablespoon, with more fat and calories than a typical hamburger.

Most parents are horrified to discover how many calories and grams of fat are in their child's favorite hamburger and fries. One Burger King Whopper with cheese contains 740 calories! Adding a regular order of fries and a large Coke brings the number of calories to over 1,100.

You may be surprised when you start comparing various options. For example, you might believe that fish is always a better choice than beef. But McDonald's Filet-O-Fish sandwich contains 370 calories and twenty-six grams of fat, compared to 255 calories and less then ten grams of fat in their regular hamburger.

Watching the fat content is the best guide to help you make a Better Bad Choice. If a Big Mac contains thirty-three grams of fat and a Wendy's cheese potato contains thirty-four grams of fat, it's a toss-up. But the Wendy's grilled chicken sandwich contains only twelve grams of fat, and would therefore be a Better Bad Choice. Remember, adding high fat condiments such as mayonnaise, cheese, and bacon will dramatically increase the fat content.

Another important fact about fast food is that most of the foods have been processed with extra ingredients. Don't assume that a chicken breast from McDonald's contains the exact same nutrient profile as a chicken breast cooked at home, unless when you cook at home you add water, flavors, dextrose, salt, chicken broth, wheat starch, thiamine hydrochloride, chicken fat, sugar, spices, calcium silicate, modified food starch, and sodium phosphate.

Making Fast Food Better Bad Choices

Smiley faces (☺) denote Better Bad Choices. There may be a few instances where the percentage of fat is around 20 percent, but I didn't award a smiley face because the calories or sodium content are too high. Many Dairy Queen desserts, for example, contain 20 percent fat or less, but five hundred or more calories. I tried to pick Better Bad Choices that are low in fat but also contain a reasonable amount of calories and sodium. In some cases, I allowed a smiley face even though the percentage of fat was higher than desirable, because the calories and grams of fat were lower than many of the other choices.

For example, the McDonald's Chicken McNuggets four-piece meal contains 54 percent fat, but it has only two hundred calories and twelve grams of fat. Because the calories and grams of fat are so much lower than many of their burgers, I rated the Chicken McNuggets four-piece meal as a Better Bad Choice. Also, a regular order of french fries is a high fat choice, but it's better than a large order of fries. Try to avoid fast food places that don't offer very many Better Bad Choices.

Remember, making Better Bad Choices also means making good choices whenever possible. Choose roast beef over burgers, because it's usually leaner. Skip the mayonnaise and cheese and you will save three hundred calories. Order low-calorie beverages, diet sodas, skim milk, or iced tea. Avoid milkshakes, malts, and regular sodas. A plain baked potato is a much better choice than French fries and it tastes even better with mustard or catsup. Catsup gives the taste of french fries and mustard makes it taste like potato salad. Carry fat-free salad dressings with you or use the ones at the restaurant; avoid the regular, high fat dressings.

The following information has been compiled from the USDA's handbook number 8 or has been supplied by the companies' own records. The USDA handbook number 8 on food compositions is available from any local government library and contains literally thousands and thousands of listings for food values. If you wish to have more information than is contained on this list, things like amino acid content, vitamin and mineral content of these foods, then contact your local government bookstore for a copy of this comprehensive food guide.

Note—Although higher in fat than 20%, the following items marked with an asterisk (*) are lower in calories than some of the higher fat choices. The following items marked with a plus (+) denote higher calories but lower fat.

Arby's

Item	Calories	Fat, g	Fat, %	Sodium, mg
Breakfast				
Apple turnover	303	18.3	54	178
Bacon and egg croissant	430	30	63	720
Blueberry turnover	320	19	53	240
Butter croissant	260	15.6	54	300
Cherry turnover	280	17.8	57	200
Ham and Swiss croissant	345	20.7	54	939
Sausage and egg croissant	519	39.2	68	632
Bacon platter	539	33	55	880
Egg platter	460	24	47	591
Ham platter	518	26.2	45	1177
Sausage platter	640	41	58	861
Bacon biscuit	318	17.9	51	904
Ham biscuit	323	16.6	46	1169
Sausage biscuit	460	31.9	62	1000
Lunch and Dinner				
Arby's Italian sub	671	38.8	52	2062
Roast beef sub	623	32	46	1847
Tuna sub	663	37	50	1342
Turkey sub*	486	19	35	2033
☺Turkey Deluxe Light Roast	260	6	21	1262
Arby's French dip	368	15.4	38	1018
Arby's French dip with cheese	429	19	40	1438
Arby's fish fillet	526	27	46	872
☺Baked potato, plain	240	1.9	7	58
Baked potato, broccoli and cheese	417	17.9	38	361
Baked potato, mushroom and cheese	515	26.7	47	923
Baked potato, sour cream and butter	463	25.2	49	203
Baked potato, deluxe	621	36.4	53	605
Chicken breast sandwich	445	22.5	45	958

Item	Calories	Fat, g	Fat, %	Sodium, mg
☺Chicken breast sandwich, roasted, deluxe light	276	7	23	777
Chicken breast sandwich, grilled, deluxe	430	19.9	42	901
Chicken breast sandwich, cordon bleu	518	27.1	47	1463
Chicken breast sandwich, grilled BBQ	386	13.1	30	1002
Croissant sandwich, mushroom and cheese	493	37.7	69	935
Croissant sandwich, ham and cheese	355	14.2	36	1400
Chicken roasted club sandwich	503	27	48	1143
☺French fries, regular*	246	13.2	48	114
French fries, cheddar	399	21.9	49	443
French fries, curly	337	17.7	47	167
☺Roast beef, junior*	233	10.8	42	519
Roast beef, regular	583	18.2	28	936
☺Roast beef, light deluxe*	294	10	31	826
Roast beef, super	552	28.3	46	1174
Cheeseburger, Bac'n Cheddar	512	31.5	55	1094
☺Chicken noodle soup	99	1.8	16	929
☺Chowder	193	10	47	1032

Salads

Item	Calories	Fat, g	Fat, %	Sodium, mg
☺Chef	205	9.5	42	796
☺Garden*	117	5.2	40	134
☺Roast chicken*	204	7.2	32	508
☺Side	25	0.3	11	30

Salad Dressings

Item	Calories	Fat, g	Fat, %	Sodium, mg
Blue cheese	295	31.2	95	489
Buttermilk ranch	349	38.5	99	471
Honey French	322	26.9	75	486
☺Light Italian*	23	1.1	43	1110
Thousand Island	298	29.2	88	493

Item	Calories	Fat, g	Fat, %	Sodium, mg
Milkshakes				
Chocolate	451	11.6	23	341
Vanilla	330	11.5	31	281
Jamocha	368	10.5	26	262

Boston Market

Item	Calories	Fat, g	Fat, %	Sodium, mg
☺Cinnamon apples	250	4.5	16	45
☺BBQ baked beans	330	9	24	630
Brownie	450	27	53	190
Caesar Salads				
Chicken	670	47	63	1860
Entree	520	43	75	1420
Side, 8 ounce	420	34	71	1120
☺Without dressing*	240	13	50	780
Chicken				
1/2 chicken with skin, 10.18 ounce	630	37	52	960
1/4 chicken, dark meat, with skin,				
4.71 ounce	330	22	61	460
☺1/4 chicken, dark meat, without skin,*				
3.71 ounce	210	10	43	320
1/4 chicken, white meat, with skin,				
5.46 ounce	330	17	45	530
☺1/4 chicken, white meat, without skin,*				
3.71 ounce	160	4	22	350
Chicken Entrees				
1/4 chicken, white meat, with cornbread,				
corn, potatoes, 15.8 ounce	690	17	22	970
1/4 chicken, white meat, with cornbread,				
cranberry, potatoes, 18.6 ounce	870	18	18	850
1/4 chicken, white meat, with cornbread,				
vegetables, corn, 15 ounce	590	15	22	910
☺1/4 chicken, white meat, with cornbread,				
vegetables, fruit, 15.3 ounce	470	11	20	790
Chicken pot pie	750	34	40	2380
Chicken salad, 3/4 cup	390	30	69	790

Item	Calories	Fat, g	Fat, %	Sodium, mg
Chicken Sandwiches				
☺Breast	420	5	11	900
☺Breast with fruit	490	6	10	910
Chunky Chicken Salad	640	31	44	1330
☺Chicken soup, 3/4 cup*	80	3	31	470
☺Soup Entree with cornbread, vegetables, potatoes	470	11	20	790
Chocolate chip cookie	340	17	44	240
Coleslaw, 3/4 cup	280	16	50	520
☺Corn, buttered	190	4	18	130
Cornbread	200	6	25	390
Cucumber salad	79	6.5	74	182
☺Fruit salad	70	0.5	7	10
Macaroni and cheese	280	10	32	760
Oatmeal raisin cookie	320	6	34	260
Pasta Salads				
☺Mediterranean	170	10	53	490
Tortellini	380	24	59	530
Potatoes				
Mashed, 2/3 cup	180	8	44	390
With gravy, 3/4 cup	200	9	40	560
☺New potatoes, 3/4 cup	140	3	18	100
☺Rice pilaf, 2/3 cup*	180	5	25	600
Spinach, creamed, 3/4 cup	300	24	73	790
☺Squash, butternut, 3/4 cup*	160	6	38	580
Stuffing, 3/4 cup	310	12	35	1140
Turkey				
☺Breast without skin, 5.07 ounce	170	1	6	850
☺Breast without skin, with gravy, 8.11 ounce	200	3.5	15	1370

Item	Calories	Fat, g	Fat, %	Sodium, mg
☺Sandwich without mayo	440	8	16	1130
Vegetable pot pie	350	12	31	1450
☺Vegetables, steamed, 2/3 cup	35	0.5	14	35
☺Zucchini with marinara, 3/4 cup*	80	4	50	470

Burger Chef

Item	Calories	Fat, g	Fat, %	Sodium, mg
Breakfast				
Apple turnover	237	9	34	N-A
Scrambled Eggs with Bacon Platter	567	31	49	1108
Scrambled Eggs with Sausage Platter	688	40	52	1411
Scrambled Eggs with Bacon Sunrise	392	21	48	978
Scrambled Eggs with Sausage Sunrise	526	33	56	1412
Breakfast Sandwich, Sausage Biscuit	418	25	54	1313
Hash browns	235	14	54	349
Lunch and Dinner				
☺Hamburger*	235	9	34	480
Cheeseburger	278	12	39	641
Double cheeseburger	402	22	49	835
Chicken club sandwich	521	25	43	N-A
Fish fillet sandwich	534	32	54	N-A
Super Chef sandwich	604	39	58	1088
Big Chef sandwich	556	36	58	840
Mushroom hamburger	520	29	50	744
Top Chef sandwich	541	33	55	1007
Funmeal feast	514	19	33	513
☺French fries, small*	204	10	44	327
French fries, large	285	14	44	456
☺Salad	11	0	0	8
Milkshakes				
Vanilla	380	10	23	325
Chocolate	403	9	20	378

Burger King

Item	Calories	Fat, g	Fat, %	Sodium, mg
Apple pie	311	14	41	412
Bacon bits	16	1	56	N-A
☺Barbecue sauce	36	0	0	397
☺Bull's-Eye barbecue sauce	22	0	0	47
Biscuit	332	17	46	754
French Toast Sticks	440	27	55	490
Scrambled egg platter	549	34	56	893
Scrambled eggs with bacon platter	610	39	58	1043
Scrambled eggs with sausage platter	768	53	62	1271
☺Bagel	272	6	20	438
Bagel with cream cheese	370	16	39	523
Bagel with bacon, egg, cheese	453	20	40	872
Bagel with egg, cheese	407	16	35	759
Bagel with ham, cheese	438	17	35	1114
Bagel with sausage, egg, cheese	626	36	52	1137
Biscuit with bacon	378	20	48	867
Biscuit with bacon, egg	467	27	52	1033
Biscuit with sausage	478	29	55	1007
Biscuit with sausage, egg	568	36	57	1172
Breakfast Buddy	255	16	56	492
Croissan'wich with bacon, egg, cheese	353	23	59	780
Croissan'wich with egg, cheese	315	20	57	607
Croissan'wich with ham, egg, cheese	351	22	56	1373
Croissan'wich with sausage, egg, cheese	534	40	67	985
American cheese	92	7	68	312
Swiss cheese	82	6	66	352
Cheeseburger, bacon double	515	31	54	748
Cheeseburger, bacon double deluxe	592	39	59	804
Cheeseburger, barbecue bacon double	536	31	52	795
Cheeseburger, deluxe	390	23	53	652

Item	Calories	Fat, g	Fat, %	Sodium, mg
Cheeseburger, double	483	27	50	851
Cheeseburger, mushroom Swiss double	473	27	51	746
☺Cheeseburger, regular*	316	15	42	651
Whopper	614	36	53	865
Whopper with cheese	706	44	56	541
Double Whopper	844	53	57	933
Double Whopper with cheese	935	24	59	1245
Whopper Jr.	380	22	52	660
☺Chicken Tenders*	236	13	50	541
Chicken sandwich, broiler	379	18	43	764
Chicken sandwich, regular	685	40	53	1417
Cream cheese	98	10	92	86
Croissant	180	10	50	285
Croutons	31	1	29	90
Apple cinnamon Danish	390	13	30	305
Cheese Danish	406	16	35	454
Cinnamon raisin Danish	449	18	36	286
Fish sandwich	495	25	45	879
French fries	372	20	48	238
☺Hamburger*	349	17	44	717
Deluxe hamburger	344	19	50	496
Regular hamburger	272	11	36	505
☺Honey Sauce	91	0	0	12
Mayonnaise	194	21	97	142
Milkshake, chocolate	326	10	28	198
Milkshake, with chocolate syrup added	409	11	24	248
Milkshake, with strawberry syrup added	394	10	23	230
Milkshake, vanilla	334	10	27	213
Blueberry muffin	292	14	43	244
Lemon poppyseed muffin	318	18	51	253
☺Mustard, per packet	2	0	0	34
☺Onion, 2.5 ounce	5	0	0	0
Onion rings	339	19	50	628

Item	Calories	Fat, g	Fat, %	Sodium, mg
☺Pickle, 5 ounce	1	0	0	119
Hash brown potatoes	213	12	51	318
Ranch Sauce	171	18	95	208
☺Chef salad without dressing*	178	9	46	568
☺Chunky Chicken Salad without dressing*	142	4	25	125
☺Garden salad without dressing*	95	5	47	125
☺Side salad without dressing	25	0	0	27
Blue cheese salad dressing	300	32	96	512
French salad dressing	290	22	68	400
Italian salad dressing, reduced calorie	170	18	95	762
Olive oil and vinegar salad dressing	310	33	96	214
Ranch salad dressing	350	37	95	316
Thousand Island salad dressing	290	26	81	403
BK Broiler Sandwich Sauce	90	10	100	95
☺Burger King AM Express	84	0	0	18
☺Sweet and sour sauce	45	0	0	52
Tartar sauce	134	14	94	202
☺Tomato	6	0	0	3

Chick-Fil-A

Item	Calories	Fat, g	Fat, %	Sodium, mg
☺Chicken sandwich*	290	9	27	870
Chicken sandwich, deluxe	300	9	27	870
☺Chicken sandwich without bun*	160	8	44	690
☺Chargrilled Chicken Sandwich	280	3	11	640
☺Chargrilled Chicken Sandwich, deluxe	290	3	10	640
☺Chargrilled Chicken Sandwich without bun*	130	3	23	630
Chargrilled Chicken Club without dressing	390	12	28	980
☺Chick-n-Strips, 4 pieces*	230	8	30	380
Chick-Fil-A Nuggets, 8 pieces	290	14	52	770
Chick-n-Q Sandwich	370	13	32	1040
☺Chicken salad sandwich	320	5	12	810
☺Chicken soup	110	1	9	760
☺Chargrilled Chicken Garden Salad	170	3	18	650
☺Chick-n-Strips Salad*	290	9	28	430
☺Chicken Salad Plate	290	5	14	570
☺Tossed salad	70	0	0	0
Coleslaw, small	130	6	38	430
☺Carrot and raisin salad, small	150	2	13	650
Waffle Potato Fries, small, salted	290	10	31	960
Icedream, small cup	350	10	26	390
☺Icedream, small cone*	140	4	25	240
Lemon Pie, per slice	280	22	71	550
Fudge nut brownie	350	16	40	650
Cheesecake, per slice	270	21	70	510

Church's Fried Chicken

Item	Calories	Fat, g	Fat, %	Sodium, mg
Apple pie	280	12.3	40	340
Biscuit	250	16.4	59	640
Chicken breast	200	12.4	56	510
Chicken breast, fried	278	17	55	560
Chicken leg	147	9	55	286
Chicken leg, boneless	140	9.1	59	160
Chicken thigh	306	22	65	448
Chicken thigh, boneless	230	16.1	63	520
Chicken wing, boneless	250	16.1	58	540
Chicken Fillet Breast	608	34	50	725
Chicken Fillet Breast with cheese	661	38	52	921
Coleslaw	92	5.5	54	230
Corn on the cob	190	5.4	26	15
Corn on the cob with butter and oil	237	9	34	65
Dessert, frozen	180	6	30	65
Fish fillet, regular	430	18	38	675
Fish fillet with cheese	483	22	41	870
French fries, large	320	16	45	185
☺French fries, regular*	210	10.5	45	60
Hot dog with cheese	330	21	57	990
Hot dog with chili	320	20	56	985
Super hot dog	520	27	47	1365
Super hot dog with cheese	580	34	53	1605
Super hot dog with chili	570	32	51	1595
Hush puppy	156	6	35	110
Okra	210	16.1	69	520
Onion rings	280	16	51	140
Mashed potatoes with gravy	90	3.3	33	520
Cajun rice	130	7	48	260

Dairy Queen

Item	Calories	Fat, g	Fat, %	Sodium, mg
Lunch and Dinner				
☺BBQ sandwich	225	4	16	250
Chicken sandwich	430	20	42	760
Chicken sandwich with cheese	480	25	47	980
☺Grilled chicken sandwich*	300	8	24	800
Chicken nuggets	276	18	59	505
Cheeseburger	365	18	44	800
Double cheeseburger	570	34	54	1070
Triple cheeseburger	820	50	55	1010
DQ Hounder	480	36	67	1800
DQ Hounder with cheese	533	40	67	1995
DQ Hounder with chili	575	41	64	1900
1/4-pound Super Dog, 7 ounce	590	38	58	1360
Super Dog, regular	280	16	51	700
Super Cheese Dog	580	34	53	1605
Super Dog with chili	570	32	50	1595
Regular hot dog with cheese	330	21	57	920
Regular hot dog with chili	320	19	53	720
Fish sandwich	370	16	39	630
Fish sandwich with cheese	420	21	45	850
☺Single hamburger*	310	13	38	580
Double hamburger	460	25	49	630
Triple hamburger	710	45	57	690
Homestyle Ultimate Hamburger	700	47	60	1110
☺French fries, small*	300	14	42	160
French fries, large	390	18	41	200
Onion rings	240	12	45	135
Desserts				
Banana split	510	11	19	250
Blizzard, Heath, regular	820	36	39	410

Item	Calories	Fat, g	Fat, %	Sodium, mg
Blizzard, Heath, small	560	23	37	280
Blizzard, strawberry, regular	740	16	19	230
Blizzard, strawberry, small	500	12	21	160
Breeze, Heath, regular	680	21	28	360
Breeze, Heath, small	450	12	24	260
☺Breeze, strawberry, regular+	590	1	1	170
☺Breeze, strawberry, small+	400	<1	2	115
Buster Bar	450	29	58	220
☺Chipper Sandwich	318	7	20	170
Dilly Bar	210	13	56	50
Double Delight	490	20	37	150
☺Float+	410	7	15	85
Freeze	500	12	21	180
Fudge Nut Bar	406	25	55	167
Mr. Misty Freeze	500	12	21	140
Mr. Misty, large+	340	trace	0	10
☺Mr. Misty, regular	250	trace	0	10
☺Mr. Misty float+	390	7	16	95
Nutty Double Fudge Sundae	580	22	34	170
Peanut Buster Parfait	710	32	40	410
QC Big Scoop, chocolate	310	14	41	100
QC Big Scoop, vanilla	300	14	42	100
Chocolate dipped cone, small	330	16	43	100
Chocolate dipped cone, large	570	24	38	145
☺Chocolate cone, regular	230	7	27	115
Chocolate cone, large	350	11	28	170
Vanilla, Queen's Choice	322	16	45	71
Vanilla, large	340	10	26	140
Vanilla, regular	230	7	27	95
☺Vanilla, small	140	4	26	60

Item	Calories	Fat, g	Fat, %	Sodium, mg
Malts				
Chocolate, large	1060	25	21	360
Chocolate, regular	760	18	21	260
Chocolate, small	520	13	22	180
Queen's Choice, vanilla, large, 21 ounce	889	21	21	304
Queen's Choice, vanilla, regular, 14.7 ounce	610	14	20	230
Milkshakes				
Chocolate, large	990	26	23	360
Chocolate, regular	540	14	23	290
☺Chocolate, small*	490	13	24	180
Queen, large	831	22	24	304
Vanilla, large	600	16	24	260
Vanilla, regular	520	14	24	240
Sundaes				
☺Chocolate, large*	440	10	20	165
☺Chocolate, regular	300	7	21	100
Strawberry, waffle cone	350	12	31	220
Yogurt, Frozen				
☺Cone, large	260	<1	3	115
☺Cone, regular	180	<1	5	80
☺Cup, large	230	<1	4	100
☺Cup, regular	170	<1	5	70
☺Strawberry sundae, regular	200	<1	4	80

Hardee's

Item	Calories	Fat, g	Fat, %	Sodium, mg
Breakfast				
Apple turnover	270	12	40	250
Big Country Breakfast with bacon	740	43	52	1800
Big Country Breakfast with ham	620	33	48	1780
Big Country Breakfast with sausage	930	61	59	2240
Egg, Biscuit, Bacon and Cheese	530	31	53	1470
Rise and Shine Biscuit	390	21	48	1000
Biscuit and gravy	510	28	49	1500
Egg and bacon with biscuit	490	27	49	1250
Bacon Biscuit	360	21	52	950
Chicken Biscuit	510	25	44	1580
Ham and Egg Biscuit	400	22	49	1600
Ham Biscuit	400	20	45	1340
Ham, Egg and Cheese Biscuit	500	27	48	1620
Canadian Sunrise Biscuit	570	32	50	1860
Cinnamon 'n' Raisin Biscuit	370	18	43	450
Country Ham Biscuit	400	20	45	1340
Sausage Biscuit	510	31	55	1360
Sausage and Egg Biscuit	560	35	56	1400
Steak Biscuit	580	32	49	1580
Steak and Egg Biscuit	550	32	52	1370
☺Three pancakes	280	2	6	890
Three pancakes with sausage	430	16	33	1290
Three pancakes with two strips of bacon	350	9	23	1130
Frisco Breakfast Ham Sandwich	460	22	43	1320
Hash browns	230	14	55	560
Lunch and Dinner				
☺Hardee's grilled chicken sandwich*	310	9	26	890
☺Hamburger	260	9	31	460

Item	Calories	Fat, g	Fat, %	Sodium, mg
Breakfast				
Cheeseburger	300	13	39	690
1/4 pound cheeseburger	470	28	54	890
Bacon cheeseburger	580	35	54	980
Big Deluxe hamburger	510	29	51	820
Big Twin hamburger	450	25	50	580
Frisco hamburger	760	50	59	1280
☺Chicken fillet sandwich*	370	13	31	1060
Grilled Chicken Frisco	620	34	49	1730
Fried chicken breast	370	15	36	1190
Fried chicken leg	170	7	37	570
☺Fried Chicken Stix, 6*	210	9	38	680
Fried Chicken Stix, 9	310	14	41	1020
Fried chicken thigh	330	15	41	1000
Fried chicken wing	200	8	36	740
Fisherman's Sandwich	480	22	41	1200
Hot dog, 4.2 ounce	300	17	51	710
Hot dog, 6.8 ounce	450	20	40	1090
Ham 'n' Cheese sandwich	530	30	51	1710
Mushroom 'n' Swiss hamburger	500	26	47	1020
☺Roast beef sandwich	270	11	37	780
Big Roast Beef sandwich	350	15	38	1080
Turkey club sandwich	390	16	37	1280
Chef salad	200	13	58	910
☺Grilled Chicken Salad*	120	4	30	520
☺Grilled Chicken and Pasta Salad	230	3	12	380
Garden salad	190	14	66	280
☺Side salad	20	0	0	20
Blue cheese salad dressing	210	18	77	790
French salad dressing, reduced calorie	130	5	35	480
House salad dressing	290	29	90	510
Italian salad dressing, reduced calorie	90	8	80	310
Thousand Island salad dressing	250	23	83	540

Item	Calories	Fat, g	Fat, %	Sodium, mg
Breakfast				
☺French fries, small*	240	10	37	100
French fries, medium	350	15	38	150
French fries, large	430	18	38	190
Crispy Curls Fries	300	16	48	840
Big French Fries	500	23	41	180
Desserts				
Blueberry muffin	400	17	38	310
Oat bran muffin	410	16	35	380
Cool Twist sundae	330	10	27	290
Cool Twist, Hot Fudge	320	10	28	260
Cool Twist, Strawberry	260	6	21	100

Jack in the Box

Item	Calories	Fat, g	Fat, %	Sodium, mg
Breakfast				
Bacon, 1 piece	35	3	77	N-A
Hash browns	160	11	62	310
Breakfast Jack	300	12	36	890
Pancake Platter	400	12	27	980
Sausage croissant	670	48	64	940
Scrambled Egg Pocket	430	21	44	1060
Supreme croissant	570	36	57	1240
Sourdough Breakfast Sandwich	380	20	47	1120
Ultimate Breakfast Sandwich	620	35	51	1800
Apple turnover	350	19	49	460
Lunch and Dinner				
☺Hamburger	280	11	35	470
Jumbo Jack	560	32	51	740
Jumbo Jack with cheese	650	40	55	1150
Grilled Sourdough Burger	670	43	58	1180
Ultimate Cheese Burger	1030	79	69	1200
1/4 pound burger	510	27	47	1080
Bacon Cheeseburger Supreme	725	46	57	1240
Cheeseburger	320	15	42	670
Double cheeseburger	450	24	48	970
Cheese nachos	570	35	55	N-A
Chicken Supreme	620	36	52	1520
Chicken sandwich	400	18	40	1290
☺Chicken Fajita Pita	290	8	25	700
Grilled Chicken Filet	430	19	40	1070
Spicy Crispy Chicken Sandwich	560	27	43	1020
Chicken Caesar Sandwich	520	26	45	1050
☺Club Pita*	280	9	29	N-A

Item	Calories	Fat, g	Fat, %	Sodium, mg
☺Taco, regular*	190	11	52	410
Taco, monster	283	17	54	760
Taco salad	380	24	57	N-A
Supreme nachos	720	41	51	N-A
☺Chicken Teriyaki Bowl	580	1.5	2	1220

Side Dishes and Finger Foods

Item	Calories	Fat, g	Fat, %	Sodium, mg
☺French fries, small	220	11	45	120
French fries, regular	350	17	44	190
French fries, jumbo	400	19	43	220
French fries, super scoop	590	29	44	330
Seasoned Curly Fries	360	20	50	1070
Onion rings	380	23	54	450
Egg rolls (3)	440	24	49	960
Egg rolls (5)	750	41	49	1640
☺Chicken strips (4)*	290	13	40	700
Chicken strips (6)	450	20	40	1100
Stuffed jalapenos (7)	420	27	58	1620
Stuffed jalapenos (10)	600	39	58	2320
Bacon & Cheddar Potato Wedges	800	58	65	1470

Milkshakes

Item	Calories	Fat, g	Fat, %	Sodium, mg
Strawberry Classic Shake	640	28	39	300
Vanilla Classic Shake	610	31	46	320
Chocolate Classic Shake	630	27	38	330
Cappuccino Classic Shake	630	29	41	320

Kentucky Fried Chicken

Item	Calories	Fat, g	Fat, %	Sodium, mg
☺Beans	132	1	14	535
☺Green beans*	36	1	27	563
Buttermilk biscuit	232	11.9	46	539
Regular biscuit	200	12	52	564
Bread sticks	110	3	25	15
Chicken Breast Center, Crispy	342	19.7	52	790
Chicken breast, Original Recipe	260	14	48	609
Chicken Breast Center, Hot & Spicy	382	25	59	905
Chicken Breast Center, Skin-free Crispy	296	16	49	435
Chicken Breast Side, Crispy	343	22.3	59	748
Chicken Breast Side, Hot & Spicy	398	27	61	922
Chicken Breast Side, Original Recipe	276	17	55	654
Chicken Breast Side, Skin-free Crispy	293	17	52	410
Dark meat, Rotisserie Gold, with skin	333	23.7	64	980
Dark meat, Rotisserie Gold, without skin	217	12.2	51	772
Drumstick, Extra Crispy	190	11	53	260
Drumstick, Hot & Spicy	190	11	53	300
Drumstick, Original Recipe	130	7	46	210
☺Drumstick, Skin-free Crispy	166	9	49	256
Hot Wings	471	33	63	1230
Spicy Chicken Bites	248	12.4	45	344
Thigh, Extra Crispy	370	25	59	540
Thigh, Hot & Spicy	370	27	65	570
Thigh, Original Recipe	260	17	58	570
Thigh, Skin-free Crispy	256	17	60	394
White meat quarter without skin or wing	335	18.7	50	1104
Wing, Extra Crispy	200	13	60	290
Wing, Hot & Spicy	210	15	62	340

Item	Calories	Fat, g	Fat, %	Sodium, mg
Wing, Original Recipe	150	8	53	380
Chicken Nuggets	46	2.9	57	140
Chicken Sandwich, Chicken Littles	169	10.1	54	331
Colonel's Chicken Sandwich	482	27.3	51	1060
☺BBQ chicken sandwich*	256	8	29	782
☺Coleslaw*	114	6	47	177
Corn on the cob	222	12	49	76
Cornbread	228	13	51	194
☺French fries, crispy*	210	11	47	493
Kentucky Fries	268	13	44	81
French fries, regular	244	11.9	44	139
Chicken gravy	59	4	61	398
Macaroni and cheese	162	8	46	531
☺Mustard Sauce*	36	0.9	23	346
Potato wedges	192	9	42	428
☺Mashed potatoes	59	trace	0	228
Mashed potatoes with gravy	109	5	41	386

Long John Silver's

Item	Calories	Fat, g	Fat, %	Sodium, mg
☺Bread sticks*	110	3	25	120
Brownie	440	22	45	150
Catfish entree	860	42	44	990
Catfish fillet	203	12	53	469
Cheesecake	120	18	52	105
☺Chicken Light Herb*	120	4	30	570
☺Chicken Plank	120	3	23	400
Chicken sandwich	280	8	26	790
☺Clam chowder with cod*	140	6	39	590
☺Clam chowder, seafood*	140	6	39	590
Clams, breaded	526	31	53	1170
☺Coleslaw*	140	6	39	260
Chocolate chip cookie	230	9	35	170
Oatmeal raisin cookie	160	10	56	150
Corn Cobbette	140	8	51	0
Fish, baked, with sauce	151	2	12	361
Fish, Batter Dipped	180	11	55	490
Fish, Crispy	150	8	48	240
Fish, Kitchen Breaded	122	5	37	374
☺Fish, Lemon Crumb	150	1	6	370
☺Fish, Light Paprika	120	<1	<7	120
Fish, Scampi Sauce	170	5	26	270
Homestyle fish sandwich	510	22	39	780
☺French fries*	220	10	41	60
☺Green beans*	20	<1	0	320
☺Honey Mustard Sauce	56	trace	0	315
Hush puppy	70	2	26	25
☺Malt vinegar	1	0	0	15
☺Mixed vegetables*	60	2	30	330
Oysters, breaded	180	9	45	195
Apple pie	320	13	37	420

Item	Calories	Fat, g	Fat, %	Sodium, mg
Cherry pie	360	13	33	200
Lemon pie	340	9	24	130
Pecan pie	446	22	44	435
Pumpkin pie	251	11	39	242
Rice pilaf	210	2	9	570
☺Roll	110	<1	<8	170
Garden salad, without dressing, with crackers	170	9	48	380
Ocean Chef Salad, without dressing, with crackers	250	9	32	1340
☺Ocean Chef Salad without dressing	110	1	8	730
☺Seafood salad without dressing	210	5	21	570
☺Seafood salad, without dressing, with crackers *	270	7	23	670
Seafood salad without dressing	380	31	73	980
☺Shrimp salad, without dressing, with crackers	183	3	15	658
Small shrimp salad without dressing	8	0	0	0
Blue cheese salad dressing	225	23	92	N-A
☺Italian salad dressing, reduced calorie*	20	1	45	882
Sea Salad salad dressing	220	21	86	N-A
Thousand Island salad dressing	225	22	88	422
Scallops, battered	159	9	51	503
Seafood gumbo with cod	120	8	60	740
☺Seafood Sauce	34	trace	0	357
Shrimp, batter dipped	30	2	60	80
Shrimp, breaded	388	23	53	1229
☺Sweet and sour sauce	20	<1	0	45
Tartar sauce	117	11	85	228

McDonald's

Item	Calories	Fat, g	Fat, %	Sodium, mg
Breakfast				
☺Egg McMuffin*	290	13	28	730
Sausage McMuffin	360	23	57	750
Sausage McMuffin with egg	440	29	59	820
☺English muffin without butter	140	2	13	220
Sausage Biscuit	430	29	61	1130
Sausage Biscuit with egg	520	35	60	1220
Bacon, Egg, Cheese Biscuit	450	27	54	1340
Biscuit	260	13	45	840
Hash brown potatoes	130	8	55	330
Hotcakes with butter and syrup	580	16	25	760
☺Hotcakes, plain	310	7	20	610
Sausage, pork	170	16	85	290
Scrambled eggs, 2	170	12	63	190
☺Cheerios	70	1	13	180
☺Wheaties	80	0	0	160
Lunch and Dinner				
Big Mac	530	28	47	960
Cheeseburger	320	14	39	750
☺Hamburger*	270	10	33	520
Quarter Pounder	420	21	45	690
Quarter Pounder with cheese	530	30	51	1160
McDonald's McChicken	510	30	53	820
☺McGrilled Chicken	260	4	14	500
☺Chicken McNuggets, 4 pieces*	200	12	54	350
Chicken McNuggets, 6 pieces	300	18	54	530
Chicken McNuggets, 9 pieces	450	27	54	800
Filet-O-Fish	360	16	40	690
☺Regular French fries*	320	10	43	135
Large fries	450	22	44	290
Super fries	540	26	43	350

Item	Calories	Fat, g	Fat, %	Sodium, mg
Salads				
☺Chef*	210	11	47	730
☺Fajita Chicken*	160	6	33	400
☺Garden*	80	4	45	60
☺Side*	45	2	40	35
Salad Dressings				
Blue cheese	190	17	80	650
Ranch	230	21	82	550
Thousand Island	190	13	61	510
☺Lite vinaigrette*	50	2	36	240
French reduced calorie	160	8	45	490
Desserts				
McDonaldland cookies	260	9	31	270
☺Low fat vanilla yogurt cone	120	0	0	85
☺Strawberry frozen yogurt sundae	40	0.1	4	115
☺Hot caramel low fat yogurt sundae	10	0.3	9	200
☺Hot fudge yogurt sundae	290	5	15	190
Nuts	40	4	90	0
Apple pie	260	13	45	200
☺Chocolate shake, small+	340	5	13	300
☺Strawberry shake, small+	340	5	13	220
☺Vanilla shake, small+	340	5	13	220
☺Fat-free apple muffin	170	0	0	200
Apple Danish	360	16	40	290
Cheese Danish	410	22	48	340
Cinnamon Danish	430	22	46	280
Raspberry Danish	400	16	36	300

Pizza Hut

Item	Calories	Fat, g	Fat, %	Sodium, mg
Beef Pizza				
☺Hand Tossed, per slice*	261	10	34	795
Pan Pizza, medium, per slice	288	18	56	675
Thick 'n' Chewy, 10-inch, 3 slices	620	20	29	N-A
Thin 'n' Crispy, 10-inch, 3 slices	490	19	35	N-A
Cheese Pizza				
☺Bigfoot, per slice*	179	5	25	959
☺Hand Tossed, medium, per slice*	253	9	32	593
Pan Pizza, medium, per slice	279	13	42	473
Thick 'n' Chewy, 10-inch, 3 slices	560	14	23	N-A
☺Thin 'n' Crispy, medium, per slice*	223	10	40	503
Thin 'n' Crispy, 10-inch, 3 slices	250	15	54	N-A
Chunky Combo Pizza				
☺Hand Tossed, medium, per slice*	280	11.6	37	823
Pan Pizza, medium, per slice	305	15.5	46	703
Thin 'n' Crispy, medium, per slice	250	12.7	46	736
Chunky Meat Pizza				
Hand Tossed, medium, per slice	325	16	44	970
Pan Pizza, medium, per slice	352	20	51	850
Thin 'n' Crispy, medium, per slice	295	17	52	882
Italian Sausage Pizza				
Hand Tossed, medium, per slice	313	15	43	871
Pan Pizza, medium, per slice	399	24	54	751
Thin 'n' Crispy, medium, per slice	282	17	54	781
Meat Lovers Pizza				
Hand Tossed, medium, per slice	321	15	42	1106

Item	Calories	Fat, g	Fat, %	Sodium, mg
Pan Pizza, medium, per slice	347	23	60	986
Thin 'n' Crispy, medium, per slice	297	16	48	1068

Pepperoni Pizza

Item	Calories	Fat, g	Fat, %	Sodium, mg
☺Bigfoot, per slice*	195	7	32	1022
Hand Tossed, medium, per slice	253	10	36	738
Pan Pizza, medium, per slice	280	18	58	618
Personal Pan Pizza, serves one	675	29	39	1335
Thick 'n' Chewy, 10-inch, 3 slices	560	18	29	N-A
☺Thin 'n' Crispy, medium, per slice*	230	11	43	678
Thin 'n' Crispy, 10-inch, 3 slices	430	17	36	N-A

Pepperoni, Mushroom, Italian Sausage Pizza

Item	Calories	Fat, g	Fat, %	Sodium, mg
☺Bigfoot, per slice*	213	9	38	1208

Pepperoni Lovers Pizza

Item	Calories	Fat, g	Fat, %	Sodium, mg
Hand Tossed, medium, per slice	335	16	43	981
Pan Pizza, medium, per slice	362	25	62	861
Thin 'n' Crispy, per slice	320	19	53	949

Pork Pizza

Item	Calories	Fat, g	Fat, %	Sodium, mg
☺Hand Tossed, per slice*	270	11	37	803
Pan Pizza, per slice	296	19	58	683
Thick 'n' Chewy, 10-inch, 3 slices	640	23	32	N-A
Thin 'n' Crispy, medium, per slice	240	12	45	713
Thin 'n' Crispy, 10-inch, 3 slices	520	23	40	N-A

Super Supreme Pizza

Item	Calories	Fat, g	Fat, %	Sodium, mg
☺Hand Tossed, medium, per slice*	276	10	33	980
Pan Pizza, medium, per slice	302	19	57	860
Thin 'n' Crispy, medium, per slice	253	12	43	700

Item	Calories	Fat, g	Fat, %	Sodium, mg
Supreme Pizza				
Hand Tossed, medium, per slice	289	12	37	894
Pan Pizza, medium, per slice	315	16	46	774
Personal Pan Pizza, serves one	647	28	39	1313
Thick 'n' Chewy, 10-inch, 3 slices	640	22	31	N-A
Thin 'n' Crispy, medium, per slice	262	14	48	819
Thin 'n' Crispy, 10-inch, 3 slices	510	21	37	N-A
Veggie Lovers Pizza				
Hand Tossed, medium, per slice	222	7	28	641

Subway

Item	Calories	Fat, g	Fat, %	Sodium, mg
Salads				
Chef, small	189	10	48	479
☺Garden, large	46	0	0	634
Ham, small	170	10	53	479
Roast beef, small	185	10	49	479
Seafood & Crab, small	198	11	50	946
Tuna, small	212	12	51	545
☺Turkey, small[*]	167	9	49	479
☺Lite Italian salad dressing, 2 tbsp.	11	0	0	475
Submarine Sandwiches				
Club, Italian, 12-inch	693	22	29	2716
Club, Italian, whole wheat, 12-inch	722	23	29	2776
Ham, 6-inch	360	11	28	839
Ham and cheese, Italian, 12-inch	643	18	25	1709
Ham and cheese, whole wheat, 12-inch	673	22	29	2508
Italian Combo, 12-inch	853	40	42	2218
Italian Combo, whole wheat, 12-inch	882	41	42	2278
Meatball, 6-inch	429	16	34	876
Meatball, Italian, 12-inch	917	44	43	2022
Meatball, whole wheat, 12-inch	947	45	43	2082
Roast beef, 6-inch	375	11	26	839
Roast beef, Italian, 12-inch	689	23	30	2287
Roast beef, whole wheat, 12-inch	717	24	30	2347
Seafood & Crab, 6-inch	388	12	28	1306
Steak, 6-inch	423	14	30	883
Steak & Cheese, Italian, 12-inch	765	32	38	1556
Steak & Cheese, whole wheat, 12-inch	711	33	42	1615
☺Subway Club, 6-inch[+][*]379	11	26	839	
☺Tuna, 6-inch[*]	402	13	29	905

Item	Calories	Fat, g	Fat, %	Sodium, mg
☺Turkey, 6-inch[*]	357	10	25	839
Turkey breast, Italian, 12-inch	645	19	27	2459
Turkey breast, whole wheat, 12-inch	674	20	27	2520
Veggie & Cheese, Italian, 12-inch	535	17	29	1076

Taco Bell

Item	Calories	Fat, g	Fat, %	Sodium, mg
Lunch and Dinner				
Bean burrito	447	14	28	1148
Beef burrito	493	21	38	1311
Beef Burrito Supreme	451	22	44	928
Cheesarito	312	13	37	451
☺Chicken Cheesarito*	334	12	32	880
Combination Cheesarito	407	16	35	1136
☺Light bean burrito	330	6	16	N-A
☺Light Burrito Supreme	350	8	20	N-A
☺Light Seven Layer*	440	9	18	N-A
MexiMelt burrito, beef	266	15	51	689
MexiMelt, chicken	257	15	52	779
Seven Layer Supreme	503	22	39	1181
☺Chicken fajita*	226	10	39	619
☺Pintos 'n' Cheese*	190	9	42	542
☺Fajita Taco, Steak*	235	11	42	507
Fajita Taco, Steak, with guacamole	269	13	43	620
Fajita Taco, Steak, with sour cream	281	15	48	507
Nachos Bellgrande	649	35	48	997
Nachos Supreme	367	27	66	471
Nachos, regular	346	18	46	399
Mexican pizza	575	37	58	1071
Salads				
Seafood salad with ranch dressing	884	66	67	1489
Seafood salad without dressing	648	42	58	917
☺Seafood salad without dressing or shell*	217	11	46	693
Taco salad	905	61	60	910
Taco salad with ranch dressing	1167	87	67	1959

Item	Calories	Fat, g	Fat, %	Sodium, mg
Taco salad without beans	822	57	62	1368
Taco salad without salsa	931	62	60	1387
Taco salad without shell	484	31	57	680
Light taco salad with chips	680	25	33	N-A
☺Light taco salad without chips*	330	9	24	N-A
Tostada, beef	322	20	56	764
☺Tostada, chicken and red sauce	264	15	51	454

Tacos

Bellgrande	335	23	62	472
☺Chicken*	171	9	47	337
☺Chicken, soft*	213	10	42	615
☺Light, Soft Taco*	180	5	25	N-A
☺Light, Soft Taco Supreme*	200	5	22	N-A
☺Light taco*	140	5	32	N-A
☺Light Taco Supreme*	160	5	28	N-A
Light Platter	1062	58	49	2068
Regular	183	11	54	276
Regular, soft	225	12	48	554
Steak, soft	218	11	45	456
Supreme	230	15	58	276
Supreme, Soft	272	16	53	554

Wendy's

Item	Calories	Fat, g	Fat, %	Sodium, mg
Breakfast				
Breakfast sandwich	370	19	46	770
Breakfast sandwich with bacon	430	23	48	1020
Breakfast sandwich with sausage	570	37	58	1175
French toast	400	19	43	850
Omelet, ham and cheese	290	21	65	570
Omelet, ham, and cheese, and mushroom	290	21	65	570
Omelet, ham, cheese, onion, and green pepper	280	19	61	485
Omelet, mushroom, green pepper, and onion	210	15	64	200
Potatoes	360	22	55	745
Sausage patty	200	18	81	405
Scrambled eggs	190	12	57	160
Lunch and Dinner				
Buns				
☺Kaiser	180	2	10	390
☺Multigrain	140	3	19	215
☺White	140	2	13	255
Cheese				
American, salad bar item	90	7	70	365
American, sandwich topping	60	6	90	295
Cheddar, shredded	110	10	82	175
Imitation, shredded	90	6	60	125
Mozzarella	90	7	70	335
Parmesan, grated	130	9	62	510
Parmesan, imitation	80	3	34	410

Item	Calories	Fat, g	Fat, %	Sodium, mg
Provolone	90	7	70	335
Swiss	90	7	70	365
Cheese sauce	39	2	46	305

Cheeseburgers

Item	Calories	Fat, g	Fat, %	Sodium, mg
Jr. Bacon, 5.5 ounce	430	25	52	840
Double	620	36	52	760
Jr., 4.4 ounce	310	13	38	770
Jr. Swiss Deluxe, 5.8 ounce	360	18	45	765
Kid's meal, 4.1 ounce	300	13	39	770

Chicken Nuggets

Item	Calories	Fat, g	Fat, %	Sodium, mg
Crispy, 6 pieces	310	21	61	660
Crispy, 9 pieces	465	32	62	990
Crispy, 20 pieces	1023	69	61	2178

Chicken Sandwiches

Item	Calories	Fat, g	Fat, %	Sodium, mg
Breast, on white bun	340	12	32	565
Club, 7.2 ounce	506	25	44	930
Fried, 6.9 ounce	440	19	39	725
Grilled, 6.2 ounce	340	13	34	815

Chili

Item	Calories	Fat, g	Fat, %	Sodium, mg
☺8 ounce*	190	6	28	670
Regular, 9 ounce	220	7	29	750
12 ounce	290	9	28	1000
Chips, cheddar	160	11	62	445
Chips, taco	260	10	35	20
Coleslaw, California	45	3	60	60
Coleslaw, salad bar item	80	5	56	165
Cookie, chocolate chip	275	13	43	256
Cottage cheese	110	4	33	425

Item	Calories	Fat, g	Fat, %	Sodium, mg
Danish				
Apple	360	14	35	380
Cheese	430	21	44	550
Cinnamon raisin	430	21	44	550
Egg, hard-cooked, salad topping	30	2	60	25
☺Fettuccine	3	14	3	
Fish sandwich, fillet, 6 ounce	460	25	49	780
French Fries				
Large	390	20	46	176
Regular	300	15	45	135
☺Small, 3.2 ounce*	240	12	45	145
Frozen Desserts				
Frosty, large	680	24	32	374
Frosty, small	400	14	32	220
Garlic toast	70	3	39	65
Hamburgers				
Big Classic on kaiser bun	470	25	48	900
Double Big Classic on kaiser bun	680	39	52	1005
Double Big Classic on white bun	560	30	48	465
Kid's meal, 3.7 ounce	260	9	31	570
Single, 1/4 pound on white bun	350	16	41	360
Single, plain, 4.4 ounce	340	15	40	500
Single, with everything	420	21	45	890
Pasta and Noodle Medley	60	2	30	5
Potatoes, Baked				
With bacon and cheese	520	18	31	1460

Item	Calories	Fat, g	Fat, %	Sodium, mg
With broccoli and cheese	400	16	36	455
With cheese	420	15	32	310
With chili and cheese	500	18	32	630
With sour cream and chives	500	23	41	135
☺Plain	270	<1	0	63
Pudding, butterscotch	90	4	40	85
Pudding, chocolate	90	4	40	70
☺Ravioli, cheese, in sauce	45	1	20	290
Refried beans	70	3	39	215
☺Rice, Spanish	70	1	13	440
☺Rotini	90	2	20	trace

Salads

Item	Calories	Fat, g	Fat, %	Sodium, mg
Caesar, side order	160	6	34	700
Chef	130	5	35	460

Whataburger

Item	Calories	Fat, g	Fat, %	Sodium, mg
Breakfast				
Potato Taquito	446	21.8	44	883
Sausage Taquito	443	25.9	53	790
Bacon Taquito	335	16.1	43	761
Egg Omelette Sandwich	288	12.8	40	602
Breakfast on a Bun	455	28.1	55	886
Breakfast on a Bun, with bacon	365	19.4	48	815
☺Three pancakes	259	5.8	20	842
Three pancakes, with sausage	426	21.1	44	1127
Hash browns	150	9	54	228
Blueberry muffin	239	7.9	29	538
Biscuit, plain	280	13.4	43	509
Biscuit with bacon	359	20.2	51	730
Biscuit with sausage	446	28.7	58	794
Biscuit with gravy	479	27.4	51	1253
Biscuit with egg and cheese	434	26.3	54	797
Biscuit with egg, cheese, bacon	511	32.9	58	1010
Biscuit with egg, cheese, sausage	601	41.6	62	1081
Breakfast Platter with sausage	785	52.7	60	1234
Breakfast Platter with bacon	695	44	57	1162
Scrambled eggs, 2	189	15	71	211
Lunch and Dinner				
Sandwiches				
Whataburger	598	26	39	1096
Whataburger Small Bun	407	18.8	41	839
Whataburger Double Meat	823	42.4	46	1298
Whataburger, Jr.	300	11.6	35	583
Justaburger	276	11.3	37	578
☺Chicken fajita*	272	6.7	22	691

Item	Calories	Fat, g	Fat, %	Sodium, mg
Beef fajita	326	11.9	33	670
Grilled chicken sandwich	442	14.2	29	1103
☺Grilled chicken sandwich, dry	385	8.5	20	989
☺Grilled chicken sandwich, dry, without bun oil or salad dressing	358	5.5	14	989
☺Grilled chicken sandwich, Small Bun, without oil, with mustard instead of salad dressing)	300	3.2	10	994
Whatachick'n Sandwich	501	23.1	41	1122

Side Orders

Item	Calories	Fat, g	Fat, %	Sodium, mg
Chicken strips, two pieces	120	5.4	40	420
☺Texas toast, per slice*	147	4.5	27	250
☺Baked potato, plain	310	0.3	8	23
Baked potato with cheese topping	510	16.3	29	636

Salads and Salad Dressings

Item	Calories	Fat, g	Fat, %	Sodium, mg
☺Garden salad	56	0	0	32
☺Grilled chicken salad	150	1.2	7	434
Thousand Island salad dressing, per packet	160	12	67	470
Ranch salad dressing, per packet	320	33	93	750
☺Lite vinaigrette salad dressing, per packet*	37	1.8	43	896

French Fries and Onion Rings

Item	Calories	Fat, g	Fat, %	Sodium, mg
☺French fries, junior*	221	12.1	49	139
French fries, regular	332	18.1	49	208
French fries, large	442	24.2	49	277
Onion rings, regular	329	19.1	52	596
Onion rings, large	493	28.7	52	893

Item	Calories	Fat, g	Fat, %	Sodium, mg
Desserts				
Apple turnover	215	10.8	45	241
Vanilla milkshake, 12 ounce	325	9.5	26	172
Strawberry milkshake, 12 ounce	352	8.9	23	168
Chocolate milkshake, 12 ounce	364	9.3	23	172
Chocolate chunk cookie	247	16	58	75
Macadamia nut cookie	269	16	53	80
Oatmeal raisin cookie	222	7	28	70
Peanut butter cookie	257	13.4	47	36

Appendix II

Better Bad Choices for Other High Fat and High Calorie Foods

Cereals

Cereals are one source of a large amount of sugar your child ingests. Notice that this table gives values for one serving of cereal. But based on what the boxes say, that could range anywhere from 3 tablespoons to 2/3 cup. Now let's be honest: when was the last time your child ate a measly 2/3 cup of cereal? Most children usually eat 2 cups or more. Here's a really quick and easy way to select a Better Bad Choice for your child's breakfast cereal.

How I Rated the Cereals

I rated these cereals based on the percentage of calories coming from sugar. If a cereal is 15% or less in sugar, I gave it a good rating. However, cereals above 15% should be considered high sugar cereals. Although most cereals don't contain much fat, they do contain a lot of sugar. And as I discussed earlier, sugar is very rapidly converted into bodyfat. Since most children love cereals, your goal should be to choose a cereal your child likes from the list of cereals below 15% sugar. If there are none that your child likes, try to select one as low as possible.

Brand	Grams sugar	Teaspoons sugar	% sugar
All Bran	6	1 1/2	30
Alpha Bits	13	3 1/4	40
Apple Jacks	14	3 1/2	51
Cap'n Crunch	12	3	44
☺Cheerios	1	1/4	3
Cinnamon Crunch	10	2 1/2	31
Cocoa Krispies	13	3 1/4	43
Cocoa Pebbles	13	3 1/4	43
Cocoa Puffs	14	3 1/2	47
☺Corn Chex	3	3/4	11
☺Corn Flakes (Kellogg's)	2	1/2	7
Count Chocula	14	3 1/2	47
100% Bran Flakes	7	1 3/4	35
Froot Loops	15	3 3/4	50
Frosted Flakes	13	3 1/4	43
Frosted Mini Wheats	12	3	27
Fruity Pebbles	12	3	48
Granola	14	3 1/2	40
☺Grape Nuts	7	1 3/4	14
Honeycomb	11	2 3/4	40
Life	10	2 1/2	33
Lucky Charms	13	3 1/4	43
☺Oatmeal	1	1/4	2
Post Fruit & Fibre	16	4	32
Post Raisin Bran	20	5	42
☺Post Toasties	2	1/2	8
☺Product 19	4	1	14
☺Puffed rice, wheat or corn	0	0	0
Raisin Bran	18	4 1/2	36
Reese's Peanut Butter Puffs	13	3 1/4	40
☺Rice Chex	2	1/2	7
☺Rice Krispies	3	3/4	10

Brand	Grams sugar	Teaspoons sugar	% sugar
☺Shredded Wheat (regular or spoon-size)	0	0	0
☺Special K	3	3/4	11
Sugar-Frosted Flakes	12	3	43
Sugar Smacks	15	3	34
☺Toasties Corn Flakes	2	1/2	8
Total	5	1 1/4	18
Trix	13	3 1/4	43
☺Wheat Chex	5	1 1/4	10
☺Wheaties	4	1	14

Candy Bars

All kids love candy and they will do anything to get it. A book about kids' nutrition wouldn't be complete without some mention of candy. Go ahead and let your child have some candy from time to time. As a nutritionist, putting together a list of candy bars that are okay to eat feels about as good as stabbing myself in the forehead with a fork. Although almost all candy is filled with sugar and fat, there are some surprising Better Bad Choices. Licorice, for example, can be a really good treat, because it's low in fat, contains a reasonable number of calories, and can easily be portion controlled.

How I Rated the Candy Bars

I looked at the combination of calories, fat, and teaspoons of sugar in each bar. In some cases, portion control is a good way to make a Better Bad Choice. Fun-size bars, for example, are smaller than the standard bar, but very satisfying. I also added some whole grain bars to the list because these present a viable option to candy bars. The asterisk denotes items that are high in fat but somewhat lower in calories than other choices.

Brand	Calories	Fat, g	Fat, %	Sugar, tsp.
3 Musketeers				
3 Musketeers bar, fun size, 2 bars*	140	4.5	29	5.5
3 Musketeers bar, miniatures, 7 pieces	170	5	26	6.75
3 Musketeers bar	260	8	27	10
Dove Chocolate				
Dove dark chocolate, 6 ounce bar	920	56	55	22
Dove dark chocolate, miniatures, 7 pieces	220	14	57	5.25
Dove dark chocolate, single bar	200	12	54	4.75
Dove milk chocolate, 6 ounce bar	920	52	51	24
Dove milk chocolate, miniatures, 7 pieces	230	13	51	6
Dove milk chocolate, single bar	200	12	54	5.25
Kudos Whole Grain Bars				
☺Low fat strawberry, single bar	90	1.5	15	2.25
☺Low fat blueberry, single bar	90	1.5	15	2.25
☺Whole grain chocolate fudge, single bar	120	4.5	22	3.25
Whole grain peanut butter, single bar	130	5	35	2.75
M&M's				
☺M&M's milk chocolate minis, single bag*	90	2.5	25	2.25
Almond, single bag	200	11	49	4.5
Peanut, king size, single bag	480	24	45	12
☺Peanut, fun size, single bag*	110	5	41	2.75
Peanut, single bag	250	13	47	6.25
☺Peanut butter, fun size, single bag*	110	6	49	2.5
Peanut butter, single bag	240	13	49	5.5
Plain, king size, single bag	440	18	37	14
☺Plain, fun size, single bag*	90	4	40	3
Plain, single bag	240	10	37	7.75

Brand	Calories	Fat, g	Fat, %	Sugar, tsp.
Mars				
Mars almond bar, fun size, 2 bars	190	10	47	5.25
Mars almond bar, single bar	240	12	45	6.5
Milky Way				
☺Milky Way, fun size, 2 bars*	180	7	35	6
Milky Way, king size, single bar	450	18	36	15.75
☺Milky Way, miniatures, 5 pieces*	190	7	33	6.5
Milky Way, single bar	280	11	35	9.25
☺Milky Way, dark, fun size, single bar*	90	3	30	3
☺Milky Way, dark, miniatures, 5 Pieces*	180	7	35	6.25
Milky Way, dark, single bar	220	8	33	7.5
Skittles				
☺Original, fun size, 3 bags	180	2	10	8
Original, king size, single bag	300	4	12	14.5
☺Original, Singles, single bag	250	3	11	11.75
☺Tropical, fun size, 2 bags	160	2	11	7.75
☺Tropical, Singles, single bag	250	3	11	11.75
☺Wild Berry, fun size, 2 bags	160	2	11	7.75
☺Wild Berry, Singles, single bag	250	3	11	11.75

Chips

Buying chips for your kids can be tricky, because some brands make misleading statements that make their chips seem better than they are. Many brands, for example, state in big bold letters that their reduced-fat chips contain 33 percent less fat than regular chips. Although they may be Better Bad Choices in some cases, they may not be your best choice. Sensibles reduced-fat BBQ potato chips contain 33 percent less fat than regular brands of BBQ chips, yet still contain 45 percent fat—just like regular Doritos Cooler Ranch chips. The best way to make a Better Bad Choice for your kids is to look at the percentage of calories from fat and forget the hype used to market the products. The list I have compiled will save you a lot of time and energy.

How I Rated the Chips

The listings below show a chip's nutritional value based on a one ounce serving, which is about ten or eleven chips. Let's face it, eating more than ten chips is no problem for most children. As you look over these values, keep a real serving size in mind and don't forget to multiply the number of servings by the calories per serving. Again, the asterisk marks items that are a little lower in calories than other choices.

Most baked chips received a Better Bad Choice rating over their fried counterparts. But sometimes baked products contain more sodium than the regular, fried chips. Tostitos baked chips, for example, contain 200 milligrams of sodium per ounce, while Doritos Cooler Ranch chips contain 170 milligrams. But because of the lower calorie and fat content, I still gave the baked chips a Better Bad Choice rating.

If you tried the lower fat chips when they first entered the market, you probably remember how bad they tasted. But time and technology have turned them into tasty treats. For starters, I suggest trying the Guiltless Gourmet nacho flavored tortilla chips. As you glance down the list, notice that reduced-fat doesn't necessarily mean low fat. Choose wisely.

Item	Calories	Fat, g	Fat, %	Sodium, mg
Combos Snacks				
Cheddar cheese crackers	150	8	48	300
Cheddar cheese pretzels	130	5	35	310
☺Nacho cheese pretzels*	130	4.5	31	320
Pepperoni and cheese pizza	140	7	45	280
☺Pizzeria pretzel*	130	4.5	31	290
Doritos				
Cooler Ranch	140	7	45	170
Dunker's	140	6	38	80
Nacho Cheesier	140	7	45	200
Nacho Cheesier reduced fat	130	5	35	210
Pizza Cravers	140	7	45	170
Taco Supreme	150	7	42	170
☺Reduced fat Cooler Ranch*	130	5	35	200
☺Reduced fat Nacho Cheesier*	130	5	35	210
Tostitos				
Bite size	140	8	51	110
100% white corn	130	6	41	80
100% white corn rounds	150	8	48	85
☺Baked	110	1	8	200
☺Baked unsalted	110	1	8	0
☺Baked Cool Ranch*	120	3	22	170
Fritos				
Chili cheese	160	10	56	260
Original	160	10	56	160
King size	160	10	56	150
Scoops	150	9	54	135
Cheetos				
Puffs	160	10	56	370
Crunchy	150	10	60	300

Item	Calories	Fat, g	Fat, %	Sodium, mg
Cheesy Chekers	150	10	60	350
Chesters popcorn (butter)	180	12	60	330
Sun Chips				
Original	140	6	38	115
French onion	140	6	38	115
Harvest Cheddar	140	6	38	115
Funyuns				
Original	140	7	45	250
Lays				
BBQ	150	10	60	220
KC Masterpiece BBQ	160	10	56	200
Potato chips	150	10	60	180
Wavy	160	10	56	120
Ranch	160	11	62	150
Sour cream	150	9	54	180
☺Baked original	110	1.5	12	150
☺Baked BBQ	110	1.5	12	220
☺Baked Masterpiece BBQ	110	1.5	12	190
☺Baked sour cream and onion	110	1.5	12	200
Ruffles				
Cheddar and sour cream	160	10	56	260
French onion	150	10	60	180
Potato chips	160	10	56	180
Masterpiece BBQ	150	9	54	190
☺Reduced fat*	140	6.7	43	130
Rold Gold				
☺Pretzels	100	0	0	420

Item	Calories	Fat, g	Fat, %	Sodium, mg
Guiltless Gourmet Baked				
☺Blue corn	110	1	8	140
☺Chili and lime	110	1	8	200
☺Ranch	110	1	8	200
☺Original	110	1	8	160
☺Original unsalted	110	1	8	26
☺Original potato chips	110	1.5	12	180
☺Original BBQ	110	1.5	12	200
☺Original sour cream and onion	110	1.5	12	200
Smart Temptations Baked				
☺Potato puffs	110	1	8	240
☺Tortilla chips	110	1	8	110
☺Unsalted tortilla chips	110	1	8	0
☺Chili lime tortilla chips	130	2.5	17	260
Sensibles (30 gram serving)				
Popcorn	150	7	42	120
†Caramel corn	120	1	7	270
BBQ reduced fat	140	7	45	180
Original reduced fat	140	7	45	140
Pringles				
BBQ	150	10	60	200
BBQ Right Crisps	140	7	45	160
BBQ Ridges	150	10	60	220
Original Ridges	150	10	60	150
Cheddar and sour cream	150	10	60	200
Cheez Ums	150	10	60	130
Ranch	150	10	60	130
Ranch Right Crisps	140	7	45	160

†Note: contains 19 grams of sugar.

Item	Calories	Fat, g	Fat, %	Sodium, mg
Chex Mix (30 gram serving)				
☺Traditional*	130	3.5	24	280
☺Cheddar*	140	4.5	29	250
Bold & Zesty	160	7	39	390
☺Hot N Spicy*	150	5	30	490
Popcorn				
☺Popcorn, air popped (unpopped, 1/4 cup)	110	1	8	10

Cookies

Let's face it, the essential ingredients in cookies are sugar and fat, which inevitably adds up to high calories. To choose Better Bad Choices, I simply listed the cookies by brand and applied the rating to the best of the bunch. I evaluated the cookies based on fat content, calories per serving, and sugar content.

How I Rated the Cookies

I gave Better Bad Choice ratings to cookies that derive less than 20 percent of their total calories from fat—with one exception. If a cookie's fat percentage was slightly higher than 20 percent but the overall calories were low, then I gave it a Better Bad Choice rating. Be sure to look at serving sizes and be honest with yourself about the amounts that your child will eat.

Brand	Calories	Fat, g	Fat, %	Sugar, tsp.
Chips Ahoy				
Chips Ahoy, regular (3 cookies)	160	7.75	44	2.5
Chips Ahoy, chunky (1 cookie)	80	4	44	1.5
Chips Ahoy, chewy (3 cookies)	170	7.75	41	3.5
Oreos				
Oreos, regular (3 cookies)	160	6.7	38	3.65
Oreos Double Stuf (2 cookies)	140	6.7	43	3.25
Newtons				
☺Apple Newtons, fat-free (2 cookies)	100	0	0	3.75
☺Strawberry Newtons, fat-free (2 cookies)	100	0	0	3.75
☺Cobbler Peach Newtons, fat-free (1 cookie)	70	0	0	2.5
Nilla Wafers				
Nilla Wafers, regular (8 cookies)	140	4.4	29	3
☺Nilla Wafers, reduced fat (8 cookies)	120	2.2	17	3
☺Nilla Wafers, chocolate (8 cookies)	110	1.7	14	3
Nabisco				
Nabisco graham, regular (2 sheets)	120	2.8	21	1.5
☺Nabisco graham, Oatmeal Crunch (2 sheets)	120	2.2	17	1.75
Nabisco graham, chocolate (2 sheets)	120	2.8	21	2
☺Nabisco graham, cinnamon (2 sheets)	120	2.2	17	2.25
☺Nabisco graham, low fat cinnamon (2 sheets)	110	1	9	2.5
☺Nabisco graham, low fat regular (2 sheets)	110	1.7	14	2
Nabisco ginger snaps (4 cookies)	120	2.8	21	2.25

Brand	Calories	Fat, g	Fat, %	Sugar, tsp.
Teddy Grahams				
Teddy Grahams, regular (24 cookies)	140	3.9	25	2
Teddy Grahams, chocolate (24 cookies)	140	4.4	29	2.25
Teddy Grahams, cinnamon (24 cookies)	140	4.4	29	2
Cameo				
Cameo, regular (2 cookies)	130	4.4	31	2.5
Nutter Butter				
Nutter Butter Bites (10 cookies)	150	6.7	40	2.25
Keebler				
Keebler vanilla wafers (8 cookies)	150	6.7	40	2.25
Keebler vanilla wafers, reduced fat (8 cookies)	130	3.3	23	2.75
Keebler Pecan Shortbread Sandies (1 cookie)	80	5	56	0.75
Keebler animals, sprinkled (6 cookies)	150	4.4	27	2.5
Keebler animals, iced (6 cookies)	150	5	30	2.25
Keebler butter, regular (5 cookies)	150	5.6	33	1.5
Keebler graham, honey (1 sheet)	140	4.4	29	1.75
Keebler graham, chocolate (1 sheet)	130	3.9	27	2.25
☺Keebler graham, Cinnamon Crisp (1 sheet)	130	2.8	19	2.25
☺Keebler graham, low fat cinnamon (1 sheet)	110	1.1	9	2.25
Sunshine				
Sunshine butter, regular (5 cookies)	140	5.6	36	1.75
Mother's				
Mother's Zoo Pals, regular (14 cookies)	140	5	32	1.5
Mother's Zoo Pals, Circus, iced (6 cookies)	140	5.6	36	3
Mother's iced with raisins (2 cookies)	180	7.8	39	3

Brand	Calories	Fat, g	Fat, %	Sugar, tsp.
Mother's butter (5 cookies)	140	5.6	36	1.25
Mother's fig bars, regular (1 cookie)	80	2.2	25	1.75
Mother's Old Fashioned sugar (2 cookies)	140	6.7	43	2
Mother's Old Fashioned chocolate chip (2 cookies)	160	7.8	44	2.75
Mother's Old Fashioned oatmeal (2 cookies)	110	5	41	2.25
Mother's Dino Grahams, regular (2 cookies)	130	3.3	23	1.75
Mother's vanilla wafers. regular (5 cookies)	140	5.6	36	3
Mother's Marias, regular (3 cookies)	170	5.6	29	2.25

Bakery Wagon

Brand	Calories	Fat, g	Fat, %	Sugar, tsp.
Bakery Wagon ginger snaps (5 cookies)	160	6.7	38	2.5

Archway

Brand	Calories	Fat, g	Fat, %	Sugar, tsp.
☺Archway fat-free cinnamon honey 3 cookies)	110	0	0	3.25
☺Archway fat-free Lemon Nuggets (4 cookies)	110	0	0	3.75
Archway regular (5 cookies)	150	5.6	33	2.75
Archway reduced fat ginger (3 cookies)	140	3.9	25	3

SnackWell

Brand	Calories	Fat, g	Fat, %	Sugar, tsp.
SnackWell chocolate chip (3 cookies)	130	3.9	27	2.5
SnackWell oatmeal raisin (2 cookies)	120	3.3	25	2.5
SnackWell peanut butter chip (3 cookies)	120	3.9	29	2.25
☺SnackWell golden devil's food (1 cookie)	50	0	0	1.75
☺SnackWell devil's food (1 cookie)	50	0	0	1.75

Brand	Calories	Fat, g	Fat, %	Sugar, tsp.
☺SnackWell chocolate sandwich*				
(2 cookies)	110	2.8	23	2.75
☺SnackWell creme sandwich*				
(2 cookies)	110	2.8	23	2.5
SnackWell double chocolate chip				
(3 cookies)	130	3.9	27	2.5

Ice Cream, Yogurt, and Sorbet

Although many of the lower fat ice creams have less fat, they also have more sugar! Nevertheless, I stuck by our basic rule and awarded Better Bad Choice ratings to items that contain less than 20 percent fat by calories, because their overall calories are lower than the premium ice creams. A good way to serve ice cream to your child is to place a small amount of fat-free or low fat ice cream in a glass and cover it with diet soda. By using different combinations of ice cream flavors and soda flavors, you can create some very interesting floats. Using a straw and a spoon is fun for kids and the foamy combination of ice cream and soda really fills them up fast. They end up satisfied with fewer calories and a lot less fat than they would get from a big bowl of ice cream.

Brand	Calories	Fat, g	Fat, %	Sugar, tsp.
Healthy Choice				
☺Bananas Foster	220	3	12	10
☺Black Forest	240	4	15	8
☺Butter Pecan Crunch	240	4	15	10.5
☺Cherry Chocolate Chunk	220	4	16	9.5
☺Chocolate Fudge Mousse	240	4	15	10
☺Cookies n Cream	240	4	15	9.5
☺Fudge Brownie	240	4	15	15
☺Fudge Brownie a la Mode	240	4	15	7.5
☺Praline & Caramel	260	4	14	12
☺Praline Caramel Cluster	260	4	14	12
☺Rocky Road	280	4	13	9.5
☺Strawberry Shortcake	240	4	15	11
☺Triple Chocolate Chunk	220	4	16	9
☺Turtle Fudge Cake	260	4	14	11.5
☺Vanilla	200	4	18	8.5
Breyers				
Butter Almond	340	22	58	7
Butter Pecan	360	24	60	7
Cherry Vanilla	300	14	42	8.5
Chocolate	320	16	45	8.5
Chocolate Chip	340	20	53	8.5
Chocolate Chip Cookie Dough	340	18	47	9.5
Cookies n Cream	340	18	47	8.5
French Vanilla	340	20	53	7.5
Fudge Twirl	320	16	45	8.5
Peach	260	12	41	8.5
Rocky Road	380	18	43	10.5
Strawberry	260	12	41	7.5
Toffee Bar Crunch	340	18	48	8.5
Vanilla	300	16	48	7.5
Vanilla/Black Cherry	300	16	48	8

Brand	Calories	Fat, g	Fat, %	Sugar, tsp.
Vanilla/Chocolate	320	16	45	8
Vanilla/Chocolate/Strawberry	300	16	48	8
Vanilla/Orange Sherbet	280	12	38	8.5

Breyers Low Fat Frozen Yogurt

Brand	Calories	Fat, g	Fat, %	Sugar, tsp.
☺Black Cherry	280	6	19	11.5
☺Chocolate	300	6	18	11
☺Chocolate Chip Cookie Dough	320	6	17	14
☺Chocolate Fudge Brownie	320	6	17	9.5
☺Peach	280	6	19	11
Strawberry	260	6	21	10.5
☺Strawberry Cheesecake	280	6	19	9.5
☺Toffee Bar Crunch	300	6	18	12
☺Vanilla	280	6	19	10.5
☺Vanilla Fudge Twirl	280	6	19	11
Vanilla Raspberry Twirl	260	6	21	11
☺Vanilla/Chocolate/Strawberry	280	6	19	10.5

Breyers Frozen Yogurt

Brand	Calories	Fat, g	Fat, %	Sugar, tsp.
Butter Pecan	340	14	37	13

Breyers Light/Reduced Fat Ice Cream

Brand	Calories	Fat, g	Fat, %	Sugar, tsp.
Brownie Marble Fudge	300	10	30	8.5
Chocolate Chocolate Chip	300	10	30	9
Chocolate Fudge Twirl	280	8	26	8.5
Fudge Toffee Parfait	300	10	30	9
Heavenly Hash	300	10	30	8
Mint Cookies n Cream	280	10	32	10
Praline Almond Crunch	280	10	32	8.5
Strawberry	240	8	30	7.5
Swiss Almond Fudge	320	12	34	8.5
Vanilla	260	9	31	7.5
Vanilla/Chocolate/Strawberry	240	8	30	7.5

Brand	Calories	Fat, g	Fat, %	Sugar, tsp.
Breyers Fat-Free Ice Cream				
☺Caramel Praline Crunch	240	0	0	9.5
☺Chocolate	190	0	0	6.5
☺Fudge Twirl	210	0	0	7.5
☺Vanilla	200	0	0	7
☺Vanilla/Strawberry	180	0	0	7
Breyers Fat-Free Frozen Yogurt				
☺Cookies n Cream	220	0	0	7.5
☺Fudge Twirl	210	0	0	7.5
☺Strawberry	190	0	0	7.5
☺Vanilla	200	0	0	7
☺Vanilla/Chocolate	200	0	0	6.5
Breyers No Sugar Added Ice Cream				
Mint Chocolate Chip	220	12	49	2.5
Vanilla	180	10	50	2
Vanilla Fudge Twirl	200	8	36	2
Vanilla/Chocolate/Strawberry	200	10	45	2
Breyers No Sugar Added Frozen Yogurt				
Vanilla	200	10	45	3
Breyers Sherbet				
☺Orange	240	2	7	9.5
☺Rainbow	240	2	7	9.5
☺Raspberry	240	2	7	10
☺Tropical	240	2	7	9.5
Breyers Viennetta				
Chocolate	380	24	57	7.5
Strawberry Frozen Yogurt	340	16	42	8
Vanilla	380	22	52	8

Brand	Calories	Fat, g	Fat, %	Sugar, tsp.
Sealtest Ice Cream				
Butter Pecan	320	18	51	6
Chocolate	280	14	45	7.5
Chocolate Chip	300	16	48	7
Chocolate Chip Cookie Dough	320	16	45	9.5
Cubic Scoops Vanilla Orange	260	8	28	8
French Vanilla	280	16	51	6.5
Fudge Royale	300	14	42	7
Heavenly Hash	300	14	42	7
Maple Walnut	320	18	51	6
Mint Chocolate Chip	300	16	48	7
Rainbow	280	14	45	6.5
Strawberry	260	12	41	7.5
Vanilla	280	14	45	6.5
Vanilla/Chocolate/Strawberry	280	12	38	7
Sealtest Gold				
Caramel Praline Almond	300	14	42	7
Cherry Chocolate Chunk	280	14	45	6
Chocolate Fudge Brownie	320	14	39	7
Neapolitan	220	12	49	4.5
Vanilla	260	14	48	5
Sealtest Fat-Free Ice Cream				
☺Chocolate	200	0	0	6.5
☺Vanilla	200	0	0	6
☺Vanilla Fudge Royale	200	0	0	6.5
☺Vanilla/Chocolate/Strawberry	200	0	0	6.5
Sealtest Low Fat Frozen Yogurt				
☺Cherry Chocolate Cordial	280	5	16	8
☺Chocolate	240	3	11	8.5

Brand	Calories	Fat, g	Fat, %	Sugar, tsp.
☺Mint Cookies in Cream	280	4	13	8.5
☺Vanilla	240	3	11	8.5

Sealtest Nonfat Frozen Yogurt

☺Black Cherry	220	0	0	8.5
☺Peach	200	0	0	8.5
☺Strawberry	200	0	0	8.5

Sealtest Sherbet

☺Orange	260	2	7	10
☺Rainbow	260	2	7	10.5

Ice Cream Bars

Brand	Calories	Fat, g	Fat, %	Sugar, tsp.
Good Humor				
☺Bubble Play Sports Bar	110	1	8	4.5
☺Calippo Cherry Bar	100	0	0	5.25
☺Calippo Grape/Lemon Bar	90	0	0	4.5
☺Chocolate Milkshake Cup	230	5	19	7.5
Classic Candy Center Crunch Bar	280	21	67	5.00
Classic Strawberry Shortcake Bar	210	11	47	5.75
Classic Toasted Almond Bar	230	11	43	6.75
Classic Chocolate Eclair Bar	220	10	41	5.5
Original Ice Cream Bar	230	13	51	6.00
Chocolate Chip Cookie Sandwich	320	15	42	8.5
☺Dinosaur Bar	110	2	16	4.25
☺First N Goal Sports Bar	90	0	0	4.5
Freeza Pizza Bar	140	5	32	4.5
☺Free Kick Sports Bar	90	0	0	4.5
Giant Vanilla Sandwich	240	10	37	5.5
Giant Neapolitan Sandwich	260	10	35	6.5
King Cone Vanilla	300	10	30	6.25
☺Hyper Stripe Bar	80	0	0	4.00
☺Jumbo Jet Star Bar	80	0	0	5.5
Reese's Peanut Butter Cup	220	16	65	4.00
☺Shoot Hoops Sports Bar	90	0	0	4.75
Sidewalk Sundae Sandwich	190	8	38	4.5
☺Snowfruit Orange Bar	140	0	0	6.25
☺Snowfruit Strawberry Bar	120	0	0	5.75
☺Snowfruit Tropical Fruit Bar	110	0	0	5.25
Snowfruit Coconut Bar	150	4	24	5.25
Watermelon Bar	80	4	40	4.00

Brand	Calories	Fat, g	Fat, %	Sugar, tsp.
Popsicle				
Creamsicle Bar	110	3	35	3.75
☺Creamsicle Frozen Yogurt Bar	100	1	9	5.5
☺Cotton Candy Bar	55	0	0	2.5
☺Fudgsicle Bar	90	1	10	3.5
☺Big Stick Cherry/Pineapple Bar	50	0	0	2.5
☺Bubble Gum Swirl Bar	55	0	0	2.5
☺Firecracker Jr. Bar	40	0	0	1.75
Vanilla Ice Cream Bar	160	11	62	3.75
☺Laser Blazer Bar	70	0	0	3.25
☺Lick-A-Color Bar	90	0	0	5.25
☺Orange Pop-Up	80	1	11	3.75
☺Rainbow Pop-Up	90	1	10	3.75
☺Rainbow Bar	90	0	0	5.25
☺Super Twin Bar, Cello	70	0	0	3.25
☺Super Twin Bar, Paper	70	0	0	3.25
Vanilla Sandwich	190	8	38	5.5
☺Supersicle Double Fudge Bar*	150	2	12	7.0
☺Supersicle Firecracker Bar	80	0	0	3.5
☺Supersicle Neon Traffic Signal Bar	80	0	0	3.5
☺Supersicle Sour Tower Bar	80	0	0	3.5
☺Supersicle Razzle Dazzle Bar	80	0	0	3.5
Klondike				
Caramel Crunch Ice Cream Bar	300	18	54	7.5
Ice Cream Kone	310	17	49	4.25
Original Ice Cream Bar	290	20	62	6.0
Krispy Ice Cream Bar	300	20	60	5.5
Krunch Bar	200	13	58	3.75
Breyers				
Breyers Cup	90	10	100	6.25
Butter Pecan Ice Cream Cone	300	17	51	5.25

Brand	Calories	Fat, g	Fat, %	Sugar, tsp.
☺Chocolate Chip Frozen Yogurt Cup	220	5	20	8.0
Vanilla Ice Cream Bar, with almonds	250	17	61	4.75
Vanilla Ice Cream Bar	230	15	58	4.75
Mint Chocolate Ice Cream Bar	230	15	59	4.75
Mint Chocolate Chip Ice Cream Cone	230	15	59	4.75
Cookie Dough Ice Cream Bar	280	17	55	6.0
Ice Cream Sandwich	250	11	39	4.5
Mini Viennetta Cappuccino/Vanilla	220	14	57	4.5
Mini Viennetta Strawberry Frozen Yogurt	185	10	48	4.0
Mini Viennetta Vanilla	220	14	57	4.5

Specialty

Brand	Calories	Fat, g	Fat, %	Sugar, tsp.
Choco Taco	320	17	48	6.75
☺Garfield Bar	90	0	0	4.25
☺Minute Maid Fruit Juicee Bar	60	0.5	7	3.0
No. 1 Bar	190	11	52	4.25
☺Screwball Cup	100	1	9	4.25
Snoopy Bar	150	8	48	4.25
☺Snow Cone	60	0	0	3.25
☺Sundae Twist Cup	160	3	17	7.25
☺Super Mario Bar	120	1	7	4.5
☺The Great White Bar	70	0	0	3.5
WWF Bar	200	10	45	4.5
X-Men Bar	140	5	32	3.0

Sealtest

Brand	Calories	Fat, g	Fat, %	Sugar, tsp.
Chip Burger Ice Cream Sandwich	320	15	42	8.5
Colonel Crunch Chocolate Eclair Bar	160	7	39	3.75
Colonel Crunch Strawberry Bar	170	8	42	3.75
Creamee Burger Ice Cream Sandwich	310	17	49	4.25
Old Nut Sundae Cone	230	9	35	5.5

Brand	Calories	Fat, g	Fat, %	Sugar, tsp.
Vanilla Flavored Ice Cream Cup	140	7	45	3.25
Chocolate Ice Cream Cup	140	7	45	3.75
Strawberry Flavored Ice Cream Cup	130	6	41	3.75
☺Orange Sherbet Cup	130	1	7	5.0
☺Fat-Free Vanilla Flavored Ice Cream Cup	100	0	0	5.0
No Sugar Added Vanilla Flavored Ice Cream Cup	90	4.5	45	1.0
Vanilla Slices	130	7	48	3.0

Eskimo Pie

Brand	Calories	Fat, g	Fat, %	Sugar, tsp.
Genuine Eskimo Pie Original	160	11	61	2.5
Milk Chocolate Coated Vanilla Bar	160	11	61	2.25
Butterscotch Crunch	170	11	58	3.5
Cherry	150	10	60	2.5
Big Bar	300	20	60	3.75
Reduced Fat Pralines n Cream	140	5	32	1.5
Reduced Fat Butter Pecan	140	7	45	1.25
☺Reduced Fat Vanilla+	110	4	32	1.5
☺Reduced Fat Fudge Ripple+	120	4	30	1.25
☺Reduced Fat Chocolate Marshmallow+	130	4	28	1.25
☺Reduced Fat Neapolitan+	110	4	32	1.5
Vanilla in Cone with Milk Chocolate and Peanuts	240	15	56	1.25
Milk Chocolate Coating with Crisped Rice	130	8	55	0.75
Dark Chocolate Coating Reduced Fat Vanilla	120	7	52	1
Sandwich Wafers Reduced Fat Vanilla	160	4	22	1

Brand	Calories	Fat, g	Fat, %	Sugar, tsp.
Weight Watchers				
☺Orange Vanilla Treat*	35	1	26	1
English Toffee Crunch Bar	110	6	49	2.5
Chocolate Treat	100	0.5	4	4.25
☺Chocolate Mousse+	40	1	22	0.75
☺Vanilla Sandwich	150	3	18	3.5
Welch's				
☺Tropical Blends Fruit Juice Bar	45	0	0	2.75
☺ Strawberry/Grape Fruit Juice Bar	25	0	0	1.5
Oreo Ice Cream Bars				
Chocolate Ice Cream	160	9	51	3.5
Vanilla Ice Cream	160	8	45	3.5
SnackWell Ice Cream Bars				
☺Low Fat Brownie Sundae Ice Cream	130	2	14	5
☺Low Fat Praline Caramel Fudge Ice Cream	140	2	13	4.5
☺Low Fat Rocky Road Ice Cream	130	2	14	4.25
☺Low Fat Vanilla Ice Cream	100	2	18	3.75
☺Low Fat Chocolate Ice Cream Sandwich	100	1.5	13	2.5
☺Low Fat Vanilla Ice Cream Sandwich	90	1.5	15	2.5
☺Low Fat Chocolate Banana Yogurt Bar	120	2	15	4.25
☺Low Fat Chocolate Cherry Yogurt Bar	120	2	15	4.25
☺Low Fat Chocolate Raspberry Yogurt Bar	120	2	15	4.25
☺Low Fat Chocolate Chocolate Yogurt Bar	120	2	15	4.25

Brand	Calories	Fat, g	Fat, %	Sugar, tsp.
Real Fruit Sorbet				
☺Chunky Cranberry Orange	100	0	0	6.25
☺Chunky Mandarin Pineapple	100	0	0	6.25
☺Chunky Lemon Peel	90	0	0	6.25
☺Chunky Mountain Strawberry	100	0	0	6.25
☺Chunky Wild Berries	100	0	0	6
☺Chunky Ruby Red Grapefruit	100	0	0	5.75
☺Chunky Georgia Peach	100	0	0	4.5
☺Chunky Tropical Blend	100	0	0	6.25
☺Chunky Red Raspberries	100	0	0	6

TCBY Frozen Yogurt

I based my Better Bad Choices for TCBY yogurt mainly on calorie content. Because most of the yogurt at TCBY is low in fat, I only selected items with less than three hundred calories per serving. And although the regular 96 percent fat-free frozen yogurt was only 20 percent fat and contained six grams of fat, I didn't select it because there are so many other lower fat and lower calorie choices.

Brand	Calories	Fat, g	Fat, %	Sugar, tsp.
Fat free giant frozen yogurt		0	0	356
Fat free super frozen yogurt	418	0	0	171
Fat free large frozen yogurt	289	0	0	118
Fat free regular. frozen yogurt	226	0	0	92
☺Fat free small frozen yogurt	162	0	0	66
☺Fat free kiddie frozen yogurt	88	0	0	36
Fat free sugar free giant	632	0	0	316
Fat free sugar free super	304	0	0	152
Fat free sugar free large	210	0	0	105
☺Fat free sugar free regular	164	0	0	82
☺Fat free sugar free small	118	0	0	59
☺Fat free sugar free kiddie	64	0	0	32
Regular, 96% fat-free giant	1027	24	21	474
Regular, 96% fat-free super	494	11	20	28
Regular, 96% fat-free large	342	8	21	156
☺Regular, 96% fat-free regular	267	6	20	126
☺Regular, 96% fat-free small	192	4	19	90
☺Regular, 96% fat-free kiddie	104	2	17	48

Meats, Poultry, and Seafood

Beef and Veal

Top round and eye of round are the lowest fat cuts of beef. I also gave a Better Bad Choice rating to a few other cuts that have a single-digit fat count. One of the best ways to serve red meat to children is to use a small portion and add plenty of their favorite vegetables, rice, potatoes, and other healthy, low fat items. Using more low fat items in a recipe reduces the overall fat content and increases the amount of fiber. Try stir-frying a small portion of red meat with a large portion of complex carbohydrates. All meats contain cholesterol, but red meats tend to have a higher saturated fat price tag. Serve red meats to your family no more than once or twice a week for optimal health.

per 3 ounce portion	Calories	Cholesterol mg	Fat g	Fat %
Beef				
Brisket	222	77	13	53
☺Chuck, arm pot roast	183	86	7	34
Chuck, blade roast	213	90	11	46
Ground beef, regular	246	76	18	66
Ground beef, lean	217	71	14	58
☺Loin, sirloin steak	165	76	6	33
Loin, tenderloin steak	179	71	9	45
Loin, top	176	65	8	41
Rib, large end roast	201	69	11	49
Rib, small end steak	188	68	10	48
☺Round, eye	143	59	4	25
Round, bottom	178	82	7	35
Round, tip roast	157	69	6	34
☺Round, top steak	153	71	4	23
Veal				
☺Cutlets	156	91	4	23
Loin chop	149	90	6	36
Rib roast	151	97	6	36
☺Shoulder, arm steak	171	132	5	26
Shoulder, blade steak	168	135	6	32

Pork and Lamb

Although the percentage of fat in pork and lamb tends to be high, I gave the Better Bad Choice rating to the cuts of meat that contain the lowest grams of fat and calories. It's important to realize that these portions are based on three ounce servings, not necessarily the serving size your child eats. A three ounce portion is about the size of a deck of cards. You can reduce the fat content further by trimming away all the visible fat before cooking. Cooked pork may be white in color, but it's definitely not as low in fat as skinless chicken or turkey breast.

per 3 ounce portion	Calories	Cholesterol mg	Fat g	Fat %
Pork				
Loin, center, chop	172	70	7	37
Loin, ribs	210	79	13	56
Loin, top chop	173	68	7	36
Loin, rib chop	186	69	8	39
Loin, sirloin roast	183	73	9	44
☺Loin, tenderloin	139	67	4	26
☺Loin, top roast*	139	66	6	39
Shoulder, blade steak	193	80	11	51
Spareribs	338	103	26	69
Lamb				
Leg, whole	162	76	7	39
Loin, chop	183	80	8	39
☺Shank, fore	159	89	5	28
Shoulder, arm chop	170	78	8	42
Shoulder, blade chop	179	78	10	50
Rib, roast	197	74	11	50

Poultry

Poultry is a good source of healthy protein if you choose the low-fat breast portions. Dark meat of poultry is high in fat: for example, chicken thighs are 54% fat. It is also important to remove the skin before cooking, because it contains deposits of pure fat. Finally, remember to handle all poultry very carefully in the kitchen and to cook it thoroughly to prevent salmonella infection.

Type per 3.5 ounce portion	Calories	Cholesterol mg	Fat g	Fat %
Chicken breast/skin	193	83	8	37
☺Chicken breast	150	74	3	18
Chicken thigh/skin	243	92	16	59
Chicken thigh	175	87	11	57
☺Turkey breast	105	46	1	9
Turkey thigh (ground)	140	61	7	45
☺Turkey breast (ground)	105	48	1	9
Goose	250	109	14.4	52
Pheasant	184	N-A	7.7	38
Quail	195	N-A	7.9	37
Duck	150	87	6.7	40

Seafood

Almost all seafood is a good choice. Just remember to feed your child cooked seafood, never raw. Children are much more susceptible than adults to food-borne illnesses. Be careful, because clams, mussels, and raw oysters may come from contaminated waters. In choosing Better Bad Choices, I mainly looked at the percentage of calories from fat and picked ones below 20 percent. Keep in mind that all shellfish is high in cholesterol. If your child has high cholesterol, limit shellfish to no more than once a week. Although catfish, salmon, and trout are high fat fish, they contain beneficial compounds, making them heart-healthy choices that can be eaten on an occasional basis.

Type per 3.5 ounce portion	Calories	Cholesterol, mg	Fat, g	Fat, %
☺Alligator	232	0	1	4
Amberjack	106	44	8	68
☺Bass, Chilean Sea	97	41	2	19
Bass, Hybrid striped	82	68	2	22
Bass, Sea	82	35	2	22
Butterfish	124	55	7	51
Carp	108	56	5	42
Catfish	140	50	9	58
☺Clams, hard shell	100	55	1.5	14
☺Cod	90	45	0.5	9
☺Crab, Blue	100	90	1	9
☺Crab, Dungeness	73	50	1	12
☺Crab, King	71	35	1	13
☺Crab, Snow	76	47	1	12
☺Crab, soft shell	63	86	1.1	16
☺Crab, Imitation	84	24	1	11
☺Crawfish	76	118	1	12
Croaker	89	52	3	30
Drum	101	54	4	36
☺Flounder	100	60	1.5	14
☺Grouper	78	31	1	12
☺Haddock	100	80	1	9
☺Hake	90	67	1	10

Type per 3.5 ounce portion	Calories	Cholesterol, mg	Fat, g	Fat, %
☺Halibut	110	35	2	16
Hoki	85	30	2	21
☺Lobster, American	80	60	0.5	6
☺Lobster, spiny	95	60	1	9
Mackerel	210	60	13	56
☺Mahi-mahi	73	62	1	12
Marlin	109	0	3	25
☺Monkfish	64	21	1	14
Mullet	99	42	3	27
☺Mussels, steamed	73	24	2	25
☺Orange Roughy	80	20	1	11
☺Oysters	70	115	1.2	15
Perch, Lake Victoria	77	76	1	12
☺Perch, Ocean	110	50	2	16
Pompano	140	43	8	51
☺Rockfish	100	40	2	18
Salmon	160	50	7	39
Salmon, Chum	130	75	4	28
Salmon, Coho	160	50	7	39
Salmon, Sockeye	180	75	9	45
☺Scallops, Bay	120	55	1	8
☺Scallops, Sea	120	55	1	8
Seatrout	88	71	3	31
☺Shark	111	42	4	32
☺Sheepshead	92	0	2	20
☺Shrimp, Black Tiger	80	160	1	11
Shrimp, Gulf	80	165	2	23
☺Shrimp, Pink	90	130	2	20
☺Shrimp, Rock	90	130	2	20
Smelt	83	60	2	22
☺Snapper	85	31	1	11
☺Sole	100	60	1.5	14

Type per 3.5 ounce portion	Calories	Cholesterol, mg	Fat, g	Fat, %
☺Squid	78	198	1	12
Sturgeon	90	0	3	30
Swordfish	130	40	4.5	31
☺Tilapia	93	55	1	10
Trout, Lake	126	49	6	43
Trout, Rainbow	140	60	6	39
☺Tuna	92	38	1	10
☺Tuna, Albacore	122	38	1.75	13
Turbot	100	0	3	27
☺Walleye	79	73	1	11
Whitefish	114	51	5	11
Whiting	110	70	3	25

About the Author

Keith Klein is the owner and CEO of the Institute of Eating Management in Houston, Texas, which specializes in designing eating management programs for athletes, obesity diabetics, and parents of overweight children. As a nutritionist, lecturer, writer, and consumer advocate devoted to educating the public about general health and nutrition, Keith offers long-term solutions, not temporary quick fixes, to people who wish to improve their appearance and health. Keith's program encompasses both physical and emotional aspects of nutrition: food science, eating management, consumer awareness, and motivation. His common-sense approach enables individuals to embark on a lifetime of healthy eating without feeling deprived.

Keith's career began in Houston during the early 1980s at the Institute of Specialized Medicine, where he designed nutritional programs for people with eating disorders, heart disease, and obesity. In 1986, he joined forces with psychiatrist John H. Simms, M.D., to develop theories on the "psychology of eating management." In 1988, Keith opened the Texas Nutrition Clinic in conjunction with Ron Preston, M.D., and the Houston Sports Medicine Clinic.

Keith has published hundreds of articles on nutrition, eating management, and food labeling. He writes columns for five magazines, and his lectures appear on both television and radio. He hosted his own national radio program, *Get Fit, Get Lean,* which aired every Saturday morning on Prime Sports Radio. He also hosts his own radio show every Saturday morning in Houston on 610 AM from 9 to10 a.m.

For the past several years, Keith has focused on deceptive food labeling. His research includes information on current labeling laws and how poorly they deliver on their promises to the consumer.

To order additional copies of

Weight Control for a Young America

Book: $16.95   Shipping/Handling: $3.50

Contact: ***BookPartners, Inc.***
P.O. Box 922
Wilsonville, OR 97070

Phone: 503-682-9821
Order: 1-800-895-7323
Fax: 503-682-8684
E-mail: bpbooks@teleport.com